atlas of
Sperm Morphology

atlas of
Sperm Morphology

Marilyn Marx Adelman, MM, MT(ASCP)

Supervisor, Serology Laboratory
Northwestern Memorial Hospital
Chicago, IL

Eileen M. Cahill, MD

Department of Pathology
Alexian Brothers Medical Center
Elk Grove Village, IL

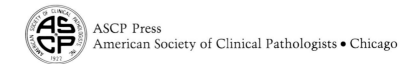
ASCP Press
American Society of Clinical Pathologists • Chicago

Cover
Nonviable spermatozoon in eosin-nigrosin viability stain.

Photographs for this presentation (Plates 1–25) were photographed on Kodak Ektachrome 50 film (tungsten) using a Zeiss brightlight photomicroscope with a Planapo 100/1.3 Oel m.1. objective, resulting in 400× magnification. Smears were examined using a brightfield microscope with a 100/1.25 oil objective. Magnifications of photographs on Plate 26 are as described.

Notice
Trade names and equipment and supplies described herein are included as suggestions only. In no way does their inclusion constitute an endorsement or preference by the American Society of Clinical Pathologists. The ASCP did not test the equipment, supplies, or procedures and, therefore, urges all readers to read and follow all manufacturers' instructions and package insert warnings concerning the proper and safe use of products.

Library of Congress Cataloging-in-Publication Data

Adelman, Marilyn Marx, 1936–
  Atlas of sperm morphology.

  Bibliography: p. 111
  Includes index.
  1. Spermatozoa—Atlases.   I. Cahill,
Eileen M., 1954–   II. Title.
QM602.A34 1989   612'.61   88-7867
ISBN 0-89189-275-3

Printed in the United States of America.

92 91 90 89   4 3 2 1

Contents

Chapter 5 Antisperm Antibodies 36

Figures

Procedures

Preface

Until now, sperm morphology has largely been taught on a face-to-face basis. Vague terminology such as "pinhead" and "amorphous form" has been used to denote the abnormal spermatozoon. No clear standardized description of "pinhead" or "amorphous form" exists. This has resulted in ambiguity and in variations in the classification of sperm aberrations by the light microscopist. Matthew Freund states in his article "Standards for the Rating of Human Sperm Morphology," which appeared in the January–March 1966 issue of the *International Journal of Fertility:* "Furthermore, the lack of an accepted manual of sperm pictures has resulted in great difficulty in teaching the rating of sperm morphology, since such teaching has had to be done on a one-to-one basis through the microscope. The difficulties encountered in teaching a personal rating system to students has led to a further proliferation of rating methods as the students become investigators and develop their own systems. In short, the rating of human sperm morphology has suffered from being subjective, qualitative, nonrepeatable, and difficult to teach to students and technicians."

The purpose of this atlas is to set forth criteria, using standard terminology based on physical characteristics of the spermatozoon as seen by the light microscopist, for the classification of sperm aberrations. These characteristics are described and pictured using color photomicrographs. The book is intended for use by physicians, technologists, and students in clinical, classroom, workshop, or office settings.

Three staining techniques have been employed.

1. Testsimplets®, a prestained, ready-for-use slide negates the need for an extensive staining set-up. It provides smears with excellent resolution that can be read within 30 minutes. Due to its simplicity, it is easily adaptable for use in the laboratory, classroom, workshop, or physician's office.

2. Papanicolaou stain provides smears that display a spectrum of color and excellent structural differentiation. This technique requires an extensive staining set-up and is most suitable for use in the clinical laboratory.

3. Hematoxylin and eosin stain provides smears with adequate resolution of detail, but not the same quality provided by the Papanicolaou or Testsimplets® preparations. This technique requires a less cumbersome staining set-up than the Papanicolaou stain and is adaptable for use in the laboratory, classroom, workshop, or physician's office.

A discussion of the male reproductive system and the process of sperm maturation has been included in this atlas to further aid and enhance the microscopist's understanding of the diagnostic significance of the procedures performed during the examination of seminal fluid. A procedure section has been included to provide a complete instructional manual on routine semen analysis.

M. Marx Adelman
E. Cahill

Acknowledgments

Our gratitude to James K. Adelman, Kenneth Bauer, PhD, Jack Garon, MD, Liliana V. Gaynor, MD, Carol Isoe, Odell Minick, Sandra Pauly, Maryann Pedone, Thelma Perez, Dolores Wainauskis, Edward Wargo, Mary Javens Wargo, and Karen Zmuda. Each had a unique role in the publication of this atlas.

The following people are responsible for the photography: Thelma Perez, electron microscopy; Marilyn Marx Adelman, sperm morphology; Eileen M. Cahill, histologic sections of the male reproductive tract.

Part One
PRINCIPLES

CHAPTER 1

Routine Semen Analysis

Spermatozoa were first seen by Leeuwenhoek and his associate, Hamm, in the 17th century. Leeuwenhoek, in a letter to the Royal Society of London in 1677 described them as "living animalcules in human semen, judging these to possess tails . . . sometimes more than a thousand were moving in an amount of material the size of a grain of sand." The following year, other scientists described spermatozoa as the "homunculus," the "little man." They conceived a completely formed little man within the sperm head, as pictured in woodcuts published in the Philosophical Transactions of the Royal Society of London (see Figure 1).

Today, semen analysis is a critical part of an infertility workup. The male is the cause of infertility in approximately 40% of infertility cases. Evaluation of seminal fluid is relatively inexpensive and easy to perform when compared with other diagnostic procedures required for an infertility workup. Therefore, semen analysis should be one of the first procedures performed. If any parameter of the semen analysis is abnormal on initial examination, it is advisable to repeat the entire analysis on 2 or 3 different specimens. Normal variation can exist and first-time collection techniques may be faulty.

Semen analysis consists of many parameters. Those most commonly evaluated during routine examination are volume, pH, viscosity, sperm density, motility, viability, and morphology. Nonroutine tests, such as the golden-hamster–egg-penetration test and hypo-osmotic swelling test, are beyond the scope of this book and are documented in other literature. Standardization of test procedures and of methods of specimen collection is imperative for obtaining valid, precise, and reproducible results.

Collection Procedures

Period of continence

The ideal period of continence (which includes abstaining from masturbation) is 48 to 72 hours. Periods of less than 48 hours can result in decreased

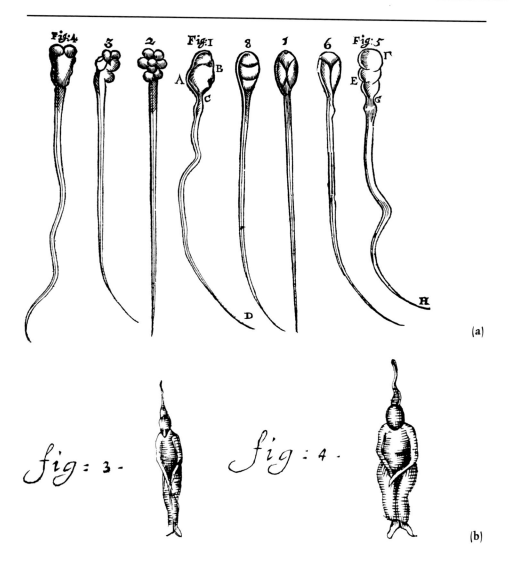

Figure 1
Two 17th Century conceptions of spermatozoa: (a) as seen by Leeuwenhoek, and (b) as tiny humans, or "homunculi."

Reprinted by permission: Volume 21 of Philosophical Transactions of the Royal Society of London.

sperm concentrations, especially in older men. Intervals that exceed 4 days result in increased sperm concentrations with a decrease in motile and viable forms.

Samples obtained at intervals congruent with each individual's natural coitus/masturbation ejaculatory pattern to obtain "average" semen values yield inconsistent results because some individuals have several ejaculations per day which deplete the supply of spermatozoa while others have only one ejaculation per month resulting in a high percentage of nonviable spermatozoa. Therefore, although this collection schedule would show the individual's average sample, it is not adequate to assess the true capacity of the male reproductive system.

Place

A sample for routine semen analysis should be obtained at the laboratory or physician's office where the analysis will be performed. If this is not possible, the specimen must be brought to the laboratory within 2 hours of collection and maintained at body temperature during transport. This can be accomplished by carrying the sample in an inside pocket or by holding it against the body with undergarments. Samples exposed to extreme heat or cold may exhibit increased viscosity and/or coagulation of the seminal fluid, resulting in a decrease in motility.

Method of collection and container

The best method for collection of seminal fluid for routine semen analysis is masturbation directly into a clean dry widemouthed glass or hard plastic container. Use of a soft plastic container may reduce the viability and motility of the spermatozoa. Care must be taken to include the entire specimen. Loss of the first portion of ejaculate may result in a decreased sperm count because this fraction normally contains the highest concentration of spermatozoa.

If split-specimen analysis is desired, 2 jars may be taped together for ease in handling. The patient is instructed to place the first fraction of ejaculate to appear into the first container and all of the remaining ejaculate into the second container. Split-specimen analysis is performed to evaluate the quality of the first portion of the ejaculate prior to dilution by seminal vesicle secretions. Split-specimen analysis is discussed further below.

Specimens obtained during coitus are usually inadequate for examination for the following reasons.

Uninterrupted coitus without condom

Upon ejaculation, semen is deposited into the vagina. At the female's midcycle spermatozoa with normal motility and morphology leave the seminal fluid, penetrate the cervical mucus within 10 minutes, and enter the cervical canal. Examination of seminal fluid remaining in the vagina will result in a decreased sperm count with a decrease in motility and an increase in abnormal forms. Semen retrieved from the vagina during nonmidcycle periods will be diluted with vaginal secretions, thereby altering results.

Uninterrupted coitus with condom

The use of the condom is contraindicated for several reasons. First, it is difficult to retrieve the entire sample from a condom, especially when the volume of seminal fluid is less than 1 mL. Specimens with volumes of less than $500\mu L$ (0.5 mL) may be totally lost or dried on the side of the condom. Second, most commercially available condoms contain spermicidal substances that result in decreased motility and viability of the spermatozoa. Two products, the Milex sheath and the Silastic seminal fluid collection device, are manufactured expressly for semen collection. They do not contain spermicidal substances. These devices do not, however, overcome the problem of specimen retrieval.

Interrupted coitus

This mode of collection is least satisfactory for two reasons. First, the sperm-rich first portion of seminal fluid may be lost if a condom is not used. Second, use of a condom is contraindicated for the reasons discussed above.

Split-Specimen Analysis

Split-specimen analysis is performed to evaluate the quality of the first portion of the ejaculate prior to dilution by the seminal vesicle secretions. Normally, the volume of the first fraction is approximately $500\mu L$ (0.5 mL). It contains the majority of the spermatozoa from the ampulla of the vas deferens and from the epididymis. Secretions from the bulbourethral and urethral glands, the vas deferens, and the prostate gland are also present. It does not contain the secretions from the seminal vesicles that are responsible for coagulation. For this reason, the first fraction normally contains a high concentration of highly motile spermatozoa in a liquid medium. This sperm-rich fraction is frequently used for artificial insemination. Therefore, results of the split specimen can be of great importance to the physician.

Approximately 6% of the time, the second fraction will contain the majority of spermatozoa. The reason for this is not completely understood. It is possible that it is due to a disorder of the nervous mechanism that controls the normal sequence of ejaculation. In these cases the second fraction is used for artificial insemination.

Characteristics of Fresh Semen

Normal semen coagulates immediately upon ejaculation due to the presence of a substrate secreted by the seminal vesicles. Secretions of the prostate gland liquefy the coagulum into a translucent, slightly viscous fluid within 5 to 25 minutes after ejaculation.

The characteristic odor of semen is similar to the odor of clorox (sodium hypochlorite). If the specimen does not possess this distinctive odor, the sample is suspect. The specimen may not have been collected properly.

The normal color of semen is light gray to white. Color variation may occur due to the presence of red blood cells, hemoglobin, and/or white blood cells produced during an inflammatory process of the male reproductive tract. It must be noted that commercially prepared dipsticks utilizing benzidine compounds to test for the presence of blood in urine give a false positive reaction for blood and/or hemoglobin in most samples of seminal fluid. This reaction cannot be explained at this time. For this reason, dipsticks must not be used to determine the presence of red blood cells and/or hemoglobin in a red- or brown-tinged semen specimen. The guaiac test may be used to make this determination (see Procedure 1.1).

Parameters of Semen Analysis

Volume

The volume of a semen sample may be measured by graduated cylinder if the quantity is sufficient or by pipet. The normal volume is considered to be 1.5 to 5.0 mL. Lower or higher volumes can reduce the fertilizing capacity of the sample. In cases of high volume, the sperm-rich first fraction can be used for artificial insemination to increase the sperm concentration by preventing dilution by the second fraction. If the sample is of low volume, the entire specimen can be used for artificial insemination to assure correct placement at the cervical os.

pH

The pH of normal semen is 7.0 to 8.3. It may be measured by pH meter if the quantity is sufficient or by dipstick.

Viscosity

Viscosity is determined by allowing the liquefied semen to drip from a pipet or pour from a container. Viscosity is considered normal when the semen conforms to the shape of its container, drips/pours easily, and is moderately viscous. The sperm count may or may not be normal in semen of normal viscosity. Semen of low viscosity conforms to the shape of its container, drips/pours easily, is watery, and has a low sperm count. Highly viscous semen may not conform to the shape of its container, does not drip/pour easily, is thick, strings out, and may not liquefy. In highly viscous semen, the sperm count may or may not be normal and motility is usually decreased.

Highly viscous specimens are difficult to handle. Sperm counts and motility vary greatly from area to area. An attempt must be made to liquefy the specimen prior to examination. One of three methods may be employed: placing the specimen on a vortex (usually yields limited results); drawing the sample up and down through a needle with a syringe to break up the coagulum; or diluting the specimen with a mucolytic agent and allowing it to stand until liquefaction occurs. Use of a mucolytic agent is the most effective method. Alevaire, the mucolytic agent of choice, is no longer available. New agents have been tested, eg, 5% solution of alpha amylase from human saliva (Sigma Chemical Corporation) in Locke's Solution (see Procedure 1.2) and Mucomyst-10 (Bristol Laboratories). These agents have proven to be satisfactory, and do not kill or immobilize the spermatozoa.

If all attempts at liquefaction fail, the results of the sperm count should be accompanied by the following statement: "Sperm density is not susceptible to precise measurement due to incomplete liquefaction of the seminal fluid." Motility can be assessed by counting motile forms in many different areas and averaging the results.

Highly viscous specimens that do not liquefy properly may be caused by any one of these three conditions: prostatic dysfunction, infection of the male reproductive tract, and the presence of sperm antibodies. The effects of these conditions on the viscosity of semen intended for insemination may be overcome by the following methods: for prostatic dysfunction, insemination with the first fraction of a split specimen, thereby eliminating the second fraction that contains the coagulating substrate; for infection, treatment of the sperm donor with antibiotics; and for the presence of antibodies, treatment with steroids and/or washing of the spermatozoa prior to insemination.

Sperm density

The sperm count is performed following complete liquefaction of the seminal fluid (see Procedure 1.3). If liquefaction does not occur, an attempt to break up the coagulum must be made utilizing techniques described in the section on viscosity. A sperm count should be performed if possible, even if attempts at liquefaction fail. In this case, results should be accompanied by the statement: "Sperm density is not susceptible to precise measurement, due to incomplete liquefaction of the seminal fluid."

The sperm count is performed with a standard Neubauer hemocytometer. The hemocytometer is divided into 2 halves. Each displays a grid that measures

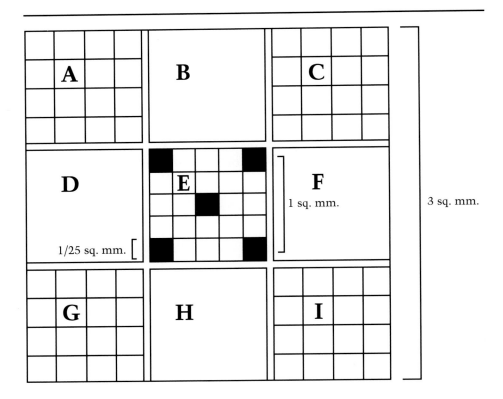

Figure 2
Standard Neubauer hemo-
cytometer.

3mm^2 by 3mm^2 (Figure 2). Each grid is divided into 9 large primary squares of 1mm^2 each (A-I). The primary center square (E) is further subdivided into 25 secondary squares of $\frac{1}{25}$ mm^2 each. The primary square E is generally utilized for counting spermatozoa. Since the depth of the hemocytometer is 0.1 mm, the count is multiplied by 10 so that final results can be expressed in mm^3.

The following guidelines may be used to determine which area of primary square E should be counted to obtain reproducible results. If more than 10 spermatozoa are present in each secondary square ($\frac{1}{25}$ mm^2), the 4 corner and center secondary squares may be counted (5 $\times$ $\frac{1}{25}$ mm^2 = $\frac{1}{5}$ mm^2). If less than 10 spermatozoa are observed per secondary square, reproducible results may be obtained by counting the spermatozoa found in all 25 secondary squares ($25 \times 1/25$ mm^2 = 1 mm^2).

If the sperm count is very low no spermatozoa may be found in primary square E. In this case the 4 corner primary squares (A, C, G, and I) (4 mm^2) or the entire grid (A-I) (9 mm^2) may be counted. The number of squares counted and the dilution can be altered until there is a satisfactory number of spermatozoa per counting area to produce a reliable count.

Sperm density is expressed as the number of spermatozoa per mL. The total number of spermatozoa present in a semen sample is equal to the number of spermatozoa per mL multiplied by the total volume of the specimen. The general formula for calculating the number of spermatozoa per mL is

Number of spermatozoa per mL
$$= 1000 \times \frac{\text{number of spermatozoa counted} \times \text{dilution} \times 10}{\text{number of mm}^2 \text{ counted}}.$$

For example: using a dilution of 1:20 and counting the spermatozoa observed in the 4 corner and center secondary squares of primary square E, the multiplication factor is 1,000,000.

Number of spermatozoa per mL
$$= 1000 \times \frac{\text{number of spermatozoa counted} \times 20 \times 10}{1/5 \text{ mm}^2}$$
$$= \text{number of spermatozoa counted} \times 1,000,000.$$

Likewise, using a dilution of 1:20 and counting all 25 secondary squares of primary square E, the multiplication factor is 200,000.

Number of spermatozoa per mL
$$= 1000 \times \frac{\text{number of spermatozoa counted} \times 20 \times 10}{1 \text{ mm}^2}$$
$$= \text{number of spermatozoa counted} \times 200,000.$$

If the seminal fluid has been diluted with a mucolytic agent to induce liquefaction, the number of spermatozoa per mL must be adjusted to account for this dilution. For example: if equal volumes of semen and mucolytic agent are mixed, the number of spermatozoa calculated per mL must be doubled.

General consensus is that 60 to 200 million spermatozoa per mL is considered to be within the normal (or average) range. Counts ranging between 40 and 60 million per mL are slightly reduced and counts of 20 to 40 million per mL, although subnormal in count, may be adequate for fertilization. Counts below 20 million per mL are considered to be subfertile. However, fertilization can still occur at this level. It should be noted that the fertilizing capacity of a semen sample is not dependent solely on the sperm count. Motility, viability, volume, and morphology are important factors and must be taken into consideration.

If no spermatozoa are found, a closer examination must be performed. The sample is centrifuged at a low speed for 10 minutes and the supernatant fluid is removed. A drop of sediment is placed on a glass slide and a coverslip placed over it. The sediment is examined for 5 minutes under 40X magnification using a light microscope for the presence of spermatozoa.

If no spermatozoa are observed in the sediment, the following procedures should be performed.

1. A fructose test (see Procedures 1.13 and 1.14).
2. An examination of postejaculatory urine for spermatozoa (see Procedure 1.15).

Fructose, a product of the seminal vesicles, provides energy for the spermatozoa. Absence of fructose in seminal fluid indicates bilateral absence of the vas deferens and/or seminal vesicles or an obstruction of the vas deferens distal to the seminal vesicles.

Spermatozoa observed in a clean voided urine specimen immediately after ejaculation indicate retrograde ejaculation.

Sperm motility

Sperm motility is considered to be the most important parameter of routine semen analysis. Samples must arrive in the laboratory within 2 hours of ejaculation because motility decreases on standing. Semen should be maintained as close to body temperature as possible. Extreme heat or cold have an adverse effect on motility. Ideally, slides for motility evaluation should be prepared and examined immediately upon complete liquefaction of the sample (see Procedure 1.4). If liquefaction does not occur, the distribution of spermatozoa and their motility ratings may be erratic. This problem can be overcome to some extent by determining the motility status of 100 spermatozoa in several different areas and averaging the results. This deviation in methodology should be noted on the final report. Sperm motility is expressed as the percentage of spermatozoa that exhibit any motion.

The quality of motility must also be determined. Motile spermatozoa may meander slowly, move with no forward progression, or exhibit straight-line, high-speed motility. The following rating system may be used to denote the quality of motility.

1+ = Spermatozoa moving but no forward progression.

2+ = Spermatozoa moving aimlessly with slow forward progression.

3+ = Spermatozoa moving at moderate speed with forward progression.

4+ = Spermatozoa moving at high speed with straight-line forward progression.

Motility slides may be left at room temperature or placed in a 37 °C incubator to approximate the temperature of the female reproductive tract. It must be noted that motility usually decreases faster at 37 °C than it does at room temperature.

Motility should be evaluated every hour for 6 hours. Agglutination of the spermatozoa may occur on standing after 1 or 2 hours. It is, therefore, important that the evaluation take more than 2 hours. Agglutination results in a reduction of motility since the spermatozoa adhere to one another in clumps. Spermatozoa may adhere to white blood cells or other debris. This should be noted on the report, but not be recorded as agglutination. Motility should be monitored the full 6 hours even though agglutination has occurred, in order to determine the status of the spermatozoa that are not agglutinated. The presence of agglutination can be indicative of an infection of the male reproductive tract and/or the presence of sperm antibodies. As discussed in the viscosity section, the methods for overcoming these two conditions are: for infection, treatment of the sperm donor with antibiotics; and for the presence of antibodies, treatment with steroids and/or washing of the spermatozoa prior to insemination. The presence of white blood cells, crystals, and/or any other debris should be noted.

Sperm motility is expressed as the percentage of spermatozoa that exhibit any motion. Quality of motility is expressed in ratings of 1+ to 4+. Sperm motility is considered to be normal if at least 60% of the spermatozoa exhibit motility ratings of 3+ or 4+.

Two investigational tests are available to measure sperm migration—the swim-up test (see Procedure 1.5) and the cervical mucus penetration test (see Procedure 1.6). The swim-up test assesses the ability of the motile spermatozoa to migrate across fluid boundaries of certain media. The cervical mucus penetration test (Penetrak, Serono) measures the distance of sperm penetration through a flat capillary tube filled with standardized estrous bovine cervical mucus in 90 minutes. Average penetration, as measured by a ruled microscope slide provided with the kit, is greater than or equal to 30 mm.

If no motility is seen, the following tests are indicated.

1. A test for sperm antibodies (see Chapter 5).

2. An examination of sperm morphology to determine midpiece or tailpiece abnormalities using stained smears as described in the section on morphology (also see Procedures 1.9–1.12).

3. A viability test (see Procedures 1.7 and 1.8).

Viability

It is important to distinguish live, immotile spermatozoa from dead spermatozoa when motility is less than 40%. Two supravital staining techniques using eosin Y are available for this determination (see Procedures 1.7 and 1.8). They are based on the principle that dead sperm cells with damaged plasma

Flow Chart
Follow-Up Clinical Procedures for Abnormal Findings.

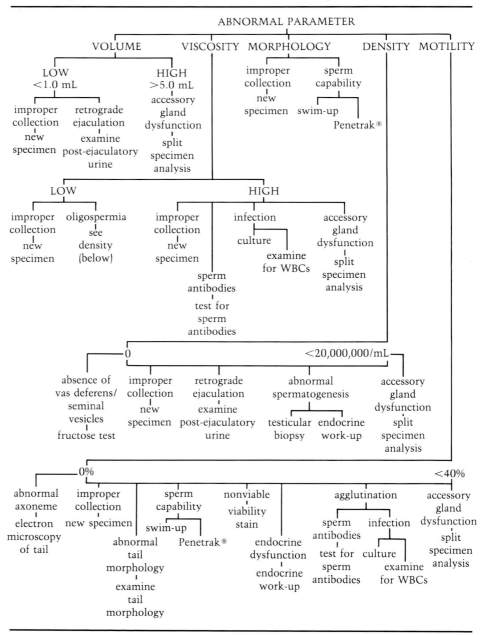

membranes will take up eosin Y stain and appear red, whereas live spermatozoa with intact membranes remain colorless. A rate of 50% or more of the spermatozoa should be viable (unstained) in a normal sperm population. A high proportion of nonmotile, viable spermatozoa may indicate structural defects of the tailpiece.

Sperm morphology

Microscopic evaluation of seminal fluid for sperm morphology is an important aspect of routine semen analysis. Identification and classification of sperm aberrations by light microscopy present a challenge to the microscopist. Details that are visible and easily defined by electron microscopy cannot be as clearly resolved in fresh preparations or on cytologically stained smears. Sperm characteristics and abnormalities are categorized in this atlas according to descriptive appearance as observed by the light microscopist.

Three staining techniques are employed (see Procedures 1.9–1.12).

1. Testsimplets®, a commercially prestained slide, ready for immediate use, is easily adaptable for office use. This slide can be read within 30 minutes.

2. Papanicolaou stain, a readily available technique, produces smears with a spectrum of color and excellent structural differentiation.

3. Hematoxylin and eosin, a readily available staining technique, produces smears with adequate resolution of detail, but not of the same quality as that of the Testsimplets® or the Papanicolaou stain.

CHAPTER 2

The Spermatozoon

The normal, mature spermatozoon is a free-swimming cell that exhibits vigorous forward motility. It consists of a flattened ovoid head that contains a nucleus with the paternal genetic material and an elongated tail for propulsion (Figure 3). The entire spermatozoon is surrounded by a cellular membrane, the plasmalemma.

Head

The normal sperm head in humans is ovoid on frontal view and pyriform when viewed laterally. It measures approximately 4 to 5 μm in length and 2 to 3 μm in width at its transverse line.

On smears stained for examination by light microscopy, the sperm head displays two distinct areas: the acrosome and the postacrosomal region. The acrosome, a caplike structure, covers the anterior two thirds of the sperm head. It contains a variety of enzymes that are released to aid the spermatozoon in penetrating the zona pellucida of the ovum. The postacrosomal region contains the nucleus, which arches up into the acrosome. The nucleus comprises approximately 65% of the sperm head.

Tailpiece

The tailpiece, approximately 50 to 55 μm in length, varies in thickness from 1 μm near the base to 0.1 μm at the tip. As revealed by electron microscopy, it is composed of an axial core complex surrounded by various sheaths. Four regions—the neckpiece, midpiece, mainpiece (principal piece), and endpiece—are defined by the nature and extent of the sheaths that surround the core complex in each section. By light microscopy, the regions can be differentiated by slight variations in the thickness of each segment.

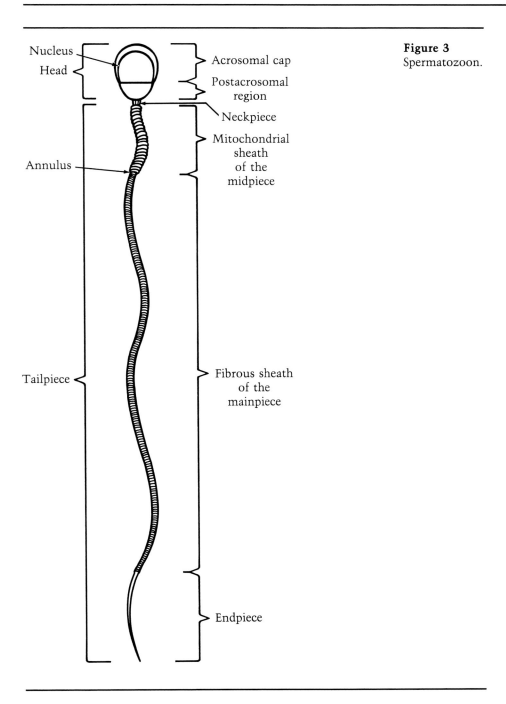

Nucleus

Head

Acrosomal cap

Postacrosomal region

Neckpiece

Mitochondrial sheath of the midpiece

Annulus

Tailpiece

Fibrous sheath of the mainpiece

Endpiece

Figure 3
Spermatozoon.

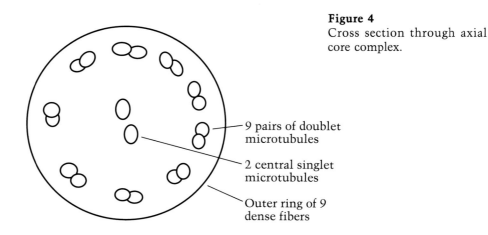

Figure 4
Cross section through axial core complex.

9 pairs of doublet microtubules

2 central singlet microtubules

Outer ring of 9 dense fibers

Electron microscopy reveals that the axial core complex consists of the axoneme, an inner core of 2 central singlet microtubules with 9 pairs of doublet microtubules arrayed around the central pair, plus an outer ring of 9 dense fibers (Figure 4).

The midpiece, connected to the head by a barely discernible neckpiece, is approximately 5 μm long and 1 μm thick. It contains the proximal portion of the axoneme, which is surrounded by 9 dense fibers. Mitochondria are wrapped in a helical arrangement around the dense outer fibers to form a sheath that produces metabolic enzymes necessary for motility. The mitochondrial sheath extends only the length of the midpiece, which terminates abruptly at the annulus, a ring of dense material fused to the plasma membrane. The annulus may prevent caudal displacement of the mitochondria.

The mainpiece, the longest portion of the tail, extends from the annulus nearly to the end of the tail. It measures approximately 45 μm in length and 0.5 μm in thickness. The 9 dense fibers of the outer ring of the midpiece gradually diminish in thickness and disappear. They extend only a few microns into the mainpiece, leaving the axoneme, surrounded by the fibrous sheath, to serve as the major portion of the tail. The fibrous sheath ends abruptly 5 to 7 μm from the tip of the tail.

The endpiece, the portion distal to the termination of the fibrous sheath, consists of the axoneme covered only by the flagellar membrane.

Spermatogenesis

Spermatogenesis, the sequence of events in which spermatogonia are transformed into mature spermatozoa, occurs in the Sertoli cells of the seminiferous tubules in the testis and in the epididymis, where the spermatozoon acquires vigorous forward motility. Complete maturation of the human spermatozoon requires approximately 74 days.

There are three principal phases.

1. Spermatocytogenesis—the process in which primitive spermatogonia type A proliferate by mitotic division to perpetuate themselves and to give rise to more highly differentiated spermatogonia type B, whose subsequent division gives rise to primary spermatocytes.

2. Meiosis—the process in which the primary spermatocyte undergoes 2 maturation divisions to reduce its chromosome number in half, so that the resulting nucleus of each gamete contains a haploid set of chromosomes.

3. Spermiogenesis—the process in which the germ cell develops a flagellum and undergoes various transformations from a spermatid to a mature spermatozoon. These transformations include elongation and flattening of the nucleus, condensation of the nucleoplasm, formation of the acrosome, and dehydration with subsequent shedding of residual cytoplasm.

CHAPTER 3

Sperm Abnormalities

Evaluation of sperm morphology is performed using a light microscope equipped with an oil objective. Stained smears are examined to determine the appearance of the spermatozoa and the presence of white blood cells, crystals, and/or other debris. Abnormal seminal fluid cytology can be classified into three categories: head anomalies, tailpiece anomalies, and immature forms.

The most frequently observed major sperm aberrations, classified on the basis of descriptive appearance as seen on stained slides, are (Figure 5):

Head anomalies

1. Vacuolation.
2. Acrosomal abnormality.
3. Bicephalic, binucleate, or paired spermatozoa.
4. Malformation of postacrosomal region (nuclear abnormality).
5. Size variation.

Tailpiece anomalies

1. Variation in length of tailpiece.
2. Lengthened neckpiece.
3. Coiled tailpiece.
4. Midpiece abnormality.
5. Cytoplasmic extrusion mass.
6. Multitailed spermatozoon.

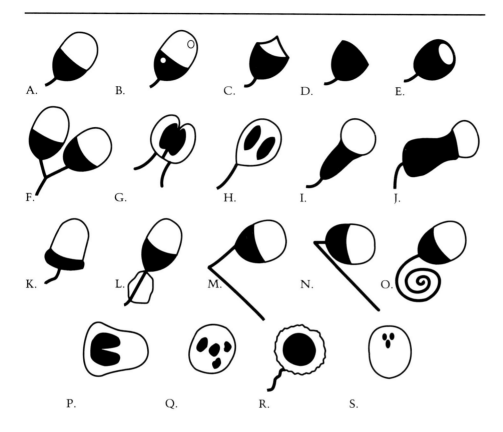

Figure 5
Sperm abnormalities (All tailpieces have been shortened).

A. Normal spermatozoon.
B. Vacuolation.
C. Acrosomal deficiency.
D. Absence of acrosome.
E. Acrosomal deficiency.
F. Bicephalic spermatozoon.
G. Paired spermatozoa due to incomplete fission during maturation.
H. Binucleate spermatozoon.
I. Elongated postacrosomal region (nuclear abnormality).
J. Elongated postacrosomal region (nuclear abnormality).
K. Flattened postacrosomal region (nuclear abnormality).
L. Normal spermatozoon with cytoplasmic extrusion mass.
M. Kinked midpiece.
N. Lengthened neckpiece.
O. Coiled tailpiece.
P. Pear-shaped immature germ cell.
Q. Immature germ cell.
R. Spermatid with tailpiece.
S. Immature germ cell.

Immature forms

1. Presence of spermatocytes.
2. Presence of spermatids.

In the discussion that follows, the capacity of abnormal spermatozoa to fertilize ova is based on in vivo observations. Abnormal spermatozoa are impeded in vivo by cervical mucus so they do not readily enter the cervical canal. Therefore, they rarely fertilize ova.

On the other hand, in vitro fertilization techniques provide a means for spermatozoa to be concentrated around the ovum, thereby increasing exposed surface area, which enhances chances for fertilization to occur. Using in vitro techniques, almost any viable spermatozoon may be capable of fertilizing ova. Therefore, unless spermatozoa are passed through mucus or other media (swim-up) prior to use, the abnormal spermatozoa will be present to fertilize ova, since natural barriers to entry are eliminated. The fact that defective gametes may unite to cause a defective fetus may account for the high rate of fetal loss through spontaneous abortion of in vitro pregnancies.

Vacuolation

Vacuoles appear as holes or bubbles in the sperm head. They occur frequently in the spermatozoa of fertile and nonfertile males and result from defects in the condensation of the nucleoplasm of the developing spermatid. Their significance in the fertilizing capacity of the spermatozoon has not been clarified.

Acrosomal abnormality

Abnormality of the acrosome most commonly presents as an acrosomal cap that occupies less than one half of the sperm head, resulting in spermatozoa that appear with rounded, pointed, or flattened-off headpieces. This defect can be termed acrosomal deficiency. In these spermatozoa the acrosome may be entirely absent, or it may manifest as a small peak on top of the nucleus or as a cap similar to an acorn cap. The acrosome contains numerous enzymes that are important in fertilization of the ovum. Deficiency in these enzymes results in decreased fertilizing capacity. On occasion, spermatozoa present with enlargement or malformation of the acrosome. Fertilizing capacity of these spermatozoa is unknown.

Bicephalic, binucleate, or paired spermatozoa

These conditions present as two-headed spermatozoa. It is not always possible to determine by light microscopy whether a spermatozoon appearing to be two-headed is bicephalic or binucleate, with one tailpiece, or whether 2 spermatozoa are paired with their tailpieces intertwined. Pairing may be caused by acrosomal deficiency, in which the spermatozoa have an affinity to pair, or by incomplete fission during spermatogenesis. Since all of these conditions render the spermatozoon abnormal, it suffices to classify them as pairing unless positive differentiation can be made. Two-headed spermatozoa are incapable of fertilization.

Malformation of postacrosomal region (nuclear abnormality)

The postacrosomal area, the cup-shaped region posterior to the acrosome, contains the nucleus, which cannot be seen by light microscopy. Aberrancies of the nucleus are presumed to cause malformations of the postacrosomal area. These spermatozoa resemble bullets, mushrooms, dumbbells, or other bizarre forms. Tapering may be associated with varicoceles. Spermatozoa exhibiting nuclear abnormalities are presumed to be incapable of fertilization in vivo.

Size variation

Sperm heads whose dimensions vary greatly from 4 to 5 μm in length and 2 to 3 μm in width at the transverse line are classified as megalospermatozoa (macrospermatozoa) if abnormally large or microspermatozoa if abnormally small. Size variation usually occurs in tandem with nuclear, acrosomal, or tailpiece anomalies. For this reason variation in sperm size results in a reduction of fertilizing capacity of the semen per unit volume.

Variation in length of tailpiece

Shortened tailpiece, demonstrated by a tailpiece considerably shorter than 55 μm, is easily recognized. This anomaly is associated with defects in which the elements of the axoneme are disordered or missing and which usually results in reduced motility. Lengthened tailpiece is an infrequent finding. Its significance is unknown.

Lengthened neckpiece

The neckpiece of the normal spermatozoon is barely discernible by light microscopy, but when abnormally lengthened the axial filament is easily identified on wet mount and on stained smear as the head is bent backward at a 90° or greater angle over the midpiece. This abnormality results in spermatozoa that propel themselves forward, dragging their poorly supported heads behind them.

Coiled tailpiece

Coiling, identified by curling of the tailpiece either below the head or encircling the entire spermatozoon, is due to an axonemal alteration in which the axial elements are disordered or missing. It is associated with reduced motility.

Midpiece abnormality

Midpiece abnormalities present as abnormal thickening or kinking in the midpiece region. This may be due to an accumulation of cytoplasmic material from the developing spermatid or disorganization of the mitochondria or midpiece elements. Midpiece abnormalities frequently occur in multitailed spermatozoa and are associated with reduced motility.

Multitailed spermatozoa

Multiple tailpieces arise from highly disorganized midpieces and neckpieces. Although usually motile, these spermatozoa are not considered to be capable of fertilization.

Cytoplasmic extrusion mass

Excess cytoplasmic material, residual from the developing spermatid, may be observed in the area of the midpiece. It frequently accompanies an elongated neckpiece. Persistence of this finding indicates poor epididymal function.

Immature forms

Developing germ cells from the meiotic and spermiogenetic phases of spermatogenesis are frequently encountered on wet preparations and on stained smears. They must be distinguished from polymorphonuclear white blood cells that may be present due to an inflammatory process of the male reproductive tract.

Polymorphonuclear leukocytes are distinctive because of their relatively regular size and characteristic nuclear properties. Their nuclei are characterized by 3 or more distinct interconnected lobes and a consistent nuclear:cytoplasmic ratio.

Spermatocytes and spermatids, in contrast to polymorphonuclear leukocytes, present in various sizes. Residual bodies and nuclei in the germ cell are not interconnected. The nuclear:cytoplasmic ratio of the dividing germ cell varies greatly in comparison with the consistent appearance of the polymorphonuclear white blood cell. Late spermatids are identified by the presence of a flagellum attached to the maturing germ cell, whose nucleus and acrosome have not fully developed.

Many aberrant spermatozoa present with more than one abnormality. Although it is feasible to calculate the percentage of each type of aberrancy observed, it is cumbersome and time consuming to report them in this manner. Since 1 anomaly renders a spermatozoon abnormal, it is expedient to derive the percentage of 200 spermatozoa that have any abnormality and to enumerate the major aberrancies seen.

The seminal fluid of fertile and nonfertile males normally contains many abnormal forms. It is generally assumed that aberrant forms are incapable of fertilization and when found in an excess of 40% can cause a reduction in the fertilizing capacity of the semen specimen. In vitro fertilization programs now in progress are expanding our understanding of the significance of morphologic abnormalities of the spermatozoon. In the near future, precise correlation of each abnormality as it relates to fertilizing ability will be achieved, perhaps necessitating a change in the morphological classification system.

CHAPTER 4

Anatomy and Histology

A basic knowledge of the anatomy of the male reproductive system (Figures 6 and 7) is useful in understanding abnormalities of semen and spermatozoa in an infertile man.

Testis

Testicular biopsies are usually done to further evaluate a man whose semen is azoospermic (no spermatozoa) or severely oligospermic (abnormally low numbers of spermatozoa) to differentiate between obstruction and abnormalities of spermatogenesis. They can provide valuable prognostic information regarding the patient's potential fertility and can help direct therapy.

Specimen handling

Testicular biopsies for infertility are usually open biopsies. Either Bouin's solution or Zenker's solution is preferred for fixation of tissue obtained because each causes less cellular shrinkage artifact than buffered formalin (see Procedures 1.16 and 1.17).

Paraffin sections should be cut to a thickness of 4 μm and stained with hematoxylin and eosin. Masson's trichrome stain may be useful for the evaluation of the tunica propria of the seminiferous tubules and also for the evaluation of Leydig cells.

Frozen sections of testicular biopsies are sometimes done prior to vasography in patients with suspected varicoceles to confirm the presence of normal spermatogenesis. Routine frozen section procedures using hematoxylin and eosin stains are usually adequate for evaluation of the testicular biopsy. Tissue imprints can be done at the time of frozen section to help evaluate the biopsy. They are prepared by lightly touching a glass slide to the surface of the tissue. Spermatozoa and germ cells will stick to the slide. The slide can then be fixed

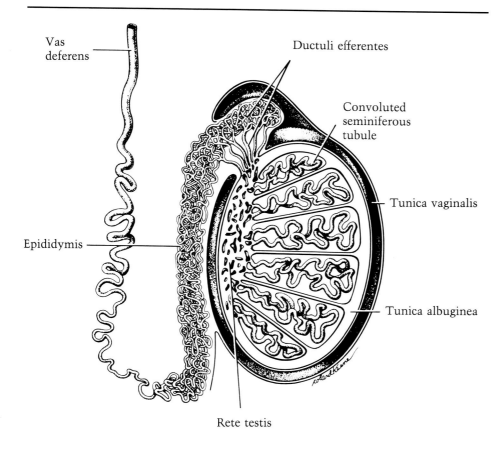

Vas deferens

Ductuli efferentes

Convoluted seminiferous tubule

Tunica vaginalis

Epididymis

Tunica albuginea

Rete testis

Figure 6
Testis and paratesticular structures.

Reprinted by permission of the publisher from *Histology: Cell and Tissue Biology* by Leon Weiss (editor), p 1002. Copyright 1983 by Elsevier Science Publishing Co., Inc.

in alcohol or formalin to be stained and evaluated with the frozen sections. The tissue sections provide information on the amount of spermatogenesis and on the morphology of the tubules, while the imprint preserves better the morphology of germ cells and of the spermatozoa. If the testicular biopsy is normal, a vasogram will be done on the patient to diagnose the presence and location of the varicocele.

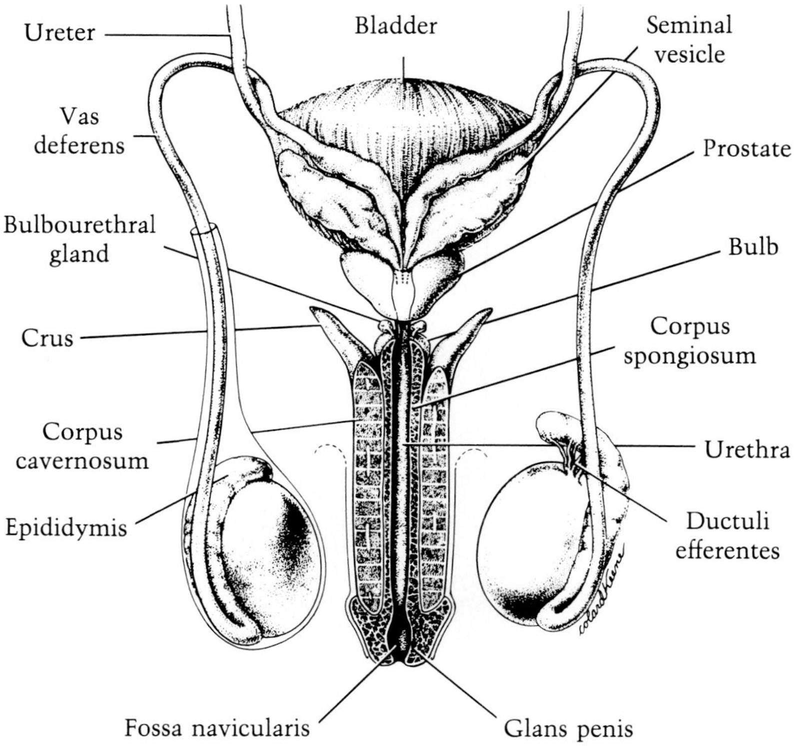

Figure 7
Male reproductive system.

Reprinted by permission of the publisher from *Histology: Cell and Tissue Biology* by Leon Weiss (editor), p 1002. Copyright 1983 by Elsevier Science Publishing Co., Inc.

Light microscopy

The seminiferous tubule is the site of spermatogenesis (Figure 6). Normal seminiferous tubules in the adult male range from 150 to 300 μm in diameter. Smaller, hypoplastic tubules usually indicate low prepubertal gonadotropin levels (hypogonadotropic hypogonadism). The tubule is surrounded by a thin layer of myoepithelial cells and an inconspicuous basement membrane. With advancing age the basement membrane thickens and focal tubular hyalinization occurs. These changes can also be seen in postpubertal gonadotropin deficiencies and in patients who have received estrogens for treatment of prostatic carcinoma. Peritubular fibrosis results from exposure to toxins, ethanol abuse, and infections, such as mumps. Oligospermia is often observed in these conditions.

The tubules are lined by Sertoli cells and germ cells. The Sertoli cells provide mechanical support and nutrition to the developing germ cells. The cell junctions between Sertoli cells form the "blood-sperm barrier." Spermatozoa are antigenic, so contact between cells of the immune system in the blood and the spermatozoa can result in production of autoantibodies. The consequences of breakdown of this barrier by infection, surgery, or trauma will be discussed later.

The germ cells develop into spermatozoa by spermatogenesis, which has already been described. A cross section of a seminiferous tubule will show germ cells in many but not all of the maturation stages, so several tubules may contain only immature germ cells, while adjacent tubules contain abundant mature spermatozoa (Plate 26:1 and 26:2). This fact becomes important in the examination of testicular biopsies. A large number of tubules must be examined before any conclusions are drawn. In the interstitium are Leydig cells (Plate 26:2) which perform the endocrine function of the testis. These cells produce androgenic steroids, including testosterone, which is required for maturation of the spermatozoa.

Abnormalities of spermatogenesis can be broken down into 3 basic groups: germ cell aplasia, germ cell hypoplasia, and maturation abnormalities. In germ cell aplasia (Sertoli-cell–only syndrome) the tubules are lined only by Sertoli cells with a complete absence of germ cells (Plate 26:3). These patients are, of course, azoospermic. Cases where a few tubules showing spermatogenesis are adjacent to tubules devoid of germ cells have also been reported. Those patients were also azoospermic. The cause can be radiation, chemotherapy (where the dose is high enough to destroy the germ cells but insufficient to damage the Sertoli cells), or exposure to toxins. Higher doses of radiation or chemotherapy will destroy the Sertoli cells as well and result in tubular sclerosis. Another primary cause is infection, eg, mumps. Fewer than one third of adult males who have had bilateral mumps orchitis will again produce semen that falls within normal parameters on analysis.

In germ cell hypoplasia, also called hypospermatogenesis, the numbers of mature spermatozoa are decreased, but the sequence of maturation is normal. The number of total germ cells may be reduced, or the numbers of immature forms may be normal, with a reduction in the number of mature spermatozoa. Some biopsies may show disorganization and sloughing of germ cells into the tubular lumen (Plate 26:4). This sloughing results in oligospermia with increased numbers of immature forms. The majority of patients have normal gonadotropin and testosterone levels, but low testosterone levels caused by renal failure, cirrhosis of the liver, or sickle cell disease may also result in germ cell hypoplasia.

Maturation arrest of the germ cells can occur at any point in the maturation sequence and results in absence or markedly decreased numbers of mature spermatozoa. It is one of the most frequent causes of infertility. A testicular biopsy will usually show failure of spermatogenesis to proceed beyond the primary or secondary spermatocyte stage. The germ cells may be increased in number and show sloughing into the tubular lumen. The tunica propria, basement membrane, Sertoli cells, and Leydig cells are normal. Many patients with hypospermatogenesis also have maturation defects, so their biopsies may show features of both. Maturation arrest is usually idiopathic but may be seen in patients with varicocele, mumps orchitis, exposure to toxic chemicals such as lead or petroleum, and in sickle cell disease. Severe oligospermia or azoospermia with increased numbers of immature forms are seen in semen analysis from these patients.

Pathologic changes due to endocrine abnormalities are discussed in other texts.

Electron microscopy

The mature spermatozoon has been described in an earlier section. Electron microscopy has no real place in routine semen analysis, but can provide additional insight into the structure of the spermatozoon. Within the head, the condensed chromatin of the nucleus and the covering acrosomal cap are revealed (Figure 8). At the center of the tail of the spermatozoon is the axoneme made up of 2 single microtubules at the core, surrounded by 9 evenly spaced doublets of microtubules (Figure 9). The axoneme extends through all of the tail and is responsible for the spermatozoon's motility. Around the outside of the microtubule doublets are 9 dense fibers (Figures 9 and 10). Sections through the midpiece of the tail show the mitochondria, which provide the energy needed to move the tail, surrounding the dense fibers (Figures 10 and 11).

Most abnormalities of spermatozoa do not require electron microscopy for detection, with one rare but noteworthy exception. Abnormalities of the axoneme are seen in immotile cilia syndromes, including Kartagener's syndrome. Immotile cilia syndrome includes a group of genetic disorders in which there is partial or total absence of the dynein arms of the microtubule doublets (Figure 9), which causes lack of motility in the cilia of the respiratory tract and abnormal or absent motility of the sperm tail. Lack of cilia motility impairs movement of mucus in the lower airways, resulting in bronchial plugging and bronchiectasis. Kartagener's syndrome defines a particular subgroup of these patients who have bronchiectasis, dextrocardia, situs inversis, and sinusitis. The typical patient with immotile cilia syndrome presents with chronic pul-

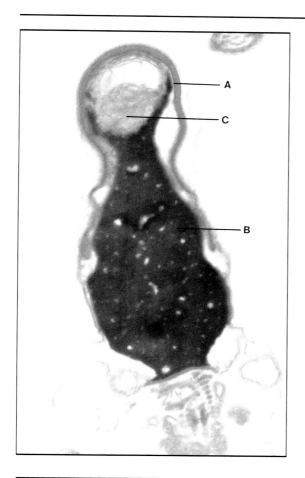

Figure 8
Head of normal spermatozoon. Note acrosomal cap (A), condensed chromatin of nucleus (B), and nuclear vacuole (C) formed during condensation of chromatin.

monary disease and bronchiectasis. The diagnosis is usually made by bronchial biopsy and electron microscopic evaluation of the cilia of the respiratory epithelial cells. Men with immotile cilia syndrome have nonmotile spermatozoa and are usually infertile.

Epididymis

The mature spermatozoa are moved by cilia in the efferent ductules to the epididymis (Figure 6), where they are stored until ejaculation (Plate 26:6). Spermatozoa from the testis are not fully mature. They are immotile and

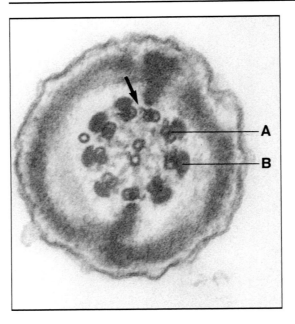

Figure 9
Cross section of sperm tail. Axoneme is made up of central pair of microtubules surrounded by 9 microtubule doublets (A) and 9 outer dense fibers (B). Note dynein arms (arrow) projecting from doublets.

cannot fertilize an ovum. They undergo capacitation and acquire motility and the ability to fertilize an ovum while in the epididymis. This process is known to be androgen-dependent but is not well understood. This fact becomes important in patients with epididymal obstruction who undergo epididymovasostomy to bypass the blockage. Some of these patients may have continued infertility due to decreased sperm motility, depending on the level of the epididymis at which the anastamosis was created. Patients with higher anastamoses have better sperm motility and better fertility than those with low anastamoses. Congenital absence of the epididymis is rare, but obstruction can follow epididymitis from chlamydia, gonorrhea, and tuberculosis infections.

From the epididymis, the spermatozoa pass through the vas deferens and the urethra during ejaculation (Figure 7).

Vas Deferens

The vas deferens is within the spermatic cord (Figure 7), which also contains nerves, arteries, and veins. It carries the mature spermatozoa from the epididymis to the urethra. Congenital atresia or absence of the vas deferens is

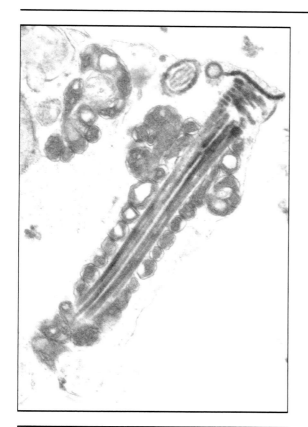

Figure 10
Longitudinal section through midpiece of tail with mitochondria.

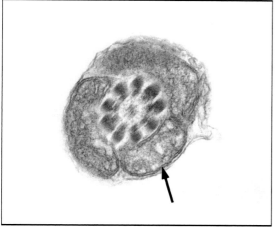

Figure 11
Cross section through midpiece of tail showing mitochondria (arrow) surrounding dense fibers.

rare. The vas deferens may be damaged during surgery, such as inguinal hernia repair, resulting in obstruction. Bilateral obstruction or congenital atresia results in azoospermia, while a unilateral obstruction can result in a low sperm count.

Varicocele

A varicocele is an enlargement of the veins of the pampiniform plexis of the spermatic cord. It is usually located in the upper part of the scrotum. Varicoceles occur in 24 to 41% of infertile men. Semen analysis will frequently show tapered spermatozoa, increased immature forms, and decreased motility; however, these features are observed with other causes of infertility and should *not* be considered pathognomonic for varicocele.

The mechanism by which a varicocele produces infertility is not clear, but may be related to increased temperature resulting from increased blood flow through the dilated veins. Varicoceles are diagnosed by vasography.

Seminal Vesicles

Spermatozoa make up only 5% of the semen. Along the way, fluids are added (see Table 1). The seminal vesicles (Figure 7) contribute a viscous yellow fluid, rich in fructose, which provides energy for the spermatozoa. This fluid constitutes 60% of the semen and provides the substrate that coagulates the semen after ejaculation. It also contains prostaglandins. The characteristics of this fluid help in ascertaining the site of obstruction in a patient with abnormal semen. If the semen is azoospermic, but contains fructose and coagulates, the obstruction is above the level of the seminal vesicles. If fructose is absent and the semen does not coagulate, there may be congenital absence of the seminal vesicles, absence of the vas deferens, or obstruction of the vas deferens distal to the seminal vesicles secondary to infection or trauma.

Prostate

The prostate contributes about 20% of the volume of the semen. Prostatic fluid is thin and watery and contains spermine phosphate and acid phosphatase (both of which are used to identify the presence of semen in medicolegal settings) as well as the proteolytic enzymes that act on the substrate from the seminal vesicles to clot, then liquefy, the semen. This fluid makes up the first fraction of the ejaculate. Prostatic dysfunction is usually a result of bacterial prostatitis and results in improper liquefaction of the semen.

Table 1
Components of Human Seminal Plasma

Component	Mean Level	Range of Values	Primary Source
Electrolytes (mg/100 mL)			
Sodium	281	240–319	
Potassium	112	56–202	
Calcium	28		Prostate
Magnesium	11		
Zinc	14	5–23	Prostate
Citric acid	376	96–1430	Prostate
Chloride	155	100–203	
Carbohydrates (mg/100 mL)			
Fructose	222	40–638	Seminal vesicles
Inositol	50	54–63	
Ascorbic acid	13		
Sorbitol	10		
Glucose	7	0–99	
Nitrogenous Compounds (mg/100 mL)			
Phosphorylcholine	315	250–380	
Spermine	273	50–350	Prostate
Urea	72		
Glycerylphosphorylcholine	66		Epididymis
Creatine	20		
Uric acid	6		
Ammonia	2		
Prostaglandins (μg/mL)			
PGE	145		Seminal vesicles
PGA	40		Seminal vesicles
PGB	21		Seminal vesicles
PGF	6		Seminal vesicles

(Continued)

Table 1 *Continued.*

Component	Mean Level	Range of Values	Primary Source
Others (mg/100 mL)			
Cholestrol	103	70–120	Prostate?
Sialic acid	124	64–219	
Glutathione	30		
Enzymes			
Acid phosphatase			Prostate
King-Armstrong units/mL	340	272–408	
Sigma U/mL	66	49–72	
Alkaline phosphatase			
Sigma U/mL	6	1–12	
Diamine oxidase			Prostate
nmoles/mL/30 mL	208		
β-Glucuronidase			
Fishman U/mL	39	26–42	
Lactic dehydrogenase			
Sigma U/mL	3808		
Leucine aminopeptidase			
Sigma U/mL	1173		Prostate
α-Amylase			
Street-Close U/100 mL/15 min	9	3–25	Prostate
Seminal proteinase (seminin, "fibrinolysin")			
μg% trypsin equivalent	30	20–50	Prostate
Total Protein (mg/100 mL)	4000	3500–5500	
Free Amino Acids (mg/100 mL)			
Neutral amino acids	638		
Basic amino acids	340		
Acidic amino acids	280		
Total	1258		

From Coffey DS. The biochemistry and physiology of the prostate and seminal vesicles. In: Walsh PC, et al, eds. *Campbell's Urology*, 5th ed., Vol. 1. Philadelphia: WB Saunders, 1986:255.

Other Seminal Fluid Components

In addition to the components of seminal fluid previously described, there are a few others which are noteworthy. The testes contribute testosterone and dihydrotestosterone, which are essential for spermatogenesis. These androgens are then taken up from the seminal fluid by the epididymis and metabolized. They help to regulate epididymal function.

The epididymis adds carnitine, acetylcarnitine, and glycerylphosphorylcholine. Their function is not clear, but they may be involved in sperm motility, since they are altered in concentration in some infertile men and in men with sperm motility defects.

In addition to acid phosphatase and spermine phosphate, the prostate produces citric acid, enzymes (see Table 1), and adds calcium to the seminal fluid. The overall composition of the prostatic fluid is alkaline. This serves to neutralize the acidic vaginal secretions and enhance sperm motility, which is optimal at a pH of 6 to 6.5.

CHAPTER 5

Antisperm Antibodies

Spermatozoa and some semen proteins are antigenic. Contact between spermatozoa and immunocompetent lymphocytes in the blood can occur if there is a breakdown of the blood-sperm barrier due to trauma, surgery, or infection. Up to 60% of men with vasectomies develop sperm-agglutinating or immobilizing antibodies. These antibodies can be detected in both serum and semen. Infertile males tend to have higher antibody levels than age-matched controls. The antibodies appear to interfere with penetration through cervical mucus and with penetration through the zona pellucida of the ovum. Women may also develop antibodies to spermatozoa. One study has linked the isoantibodies that women develop with the autoimmune antibodies of their spouses. These antibodies may be specific to an individual or may react with all human spermatozoa (Figure 12).

The variety of tests available to detect antibodies to spermatozoa is beyond the scope of this text. Immunofluorescence techniques to identify the part of the spermatozoa to which the antibody was directed were used in the past but have been replaced by hemagglutination, hemadsorption, ELISA (enzyme-linked immunosorbent assay) (Universal Diagnostic Systems) and immunobead techniques. Sperm agglutination tests (SAT) and sperm immobilization tests (SIT) are the oldest methods for determining the presence of antisperm antibodies and are still the standards to which all other tests are compared.

The role of antisperm antibodies in causing infertility is not completely understood. It has been demonstrated that autoantibodies and isoantibodies interfere with sperm motility and penetration of the cervical mucus and the zona pellucida. Immune deposits have also been found surrounding the seminiferous tubules and in the germ cells of some infertile males. These men also had serum autoantibodies to spermatozoa.

Treatment with steroids and other immuno-suppressive drugs can improve fertility in patients with antisperm antibodies.

The causes of male infertility are still poorly understood, but careful evaluation, including a good history and physical examination, laboratory studies

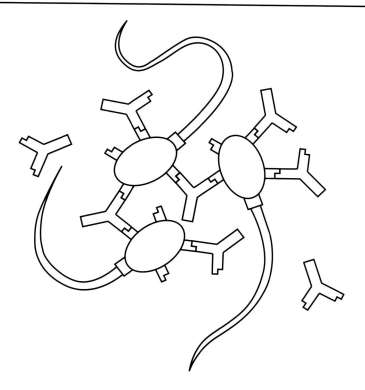

Figure 12
Spermatozoa agglutinated by
autoantibodies binding to
antigens on cell surface. They
may agglutinate head to head
or tail to tail.

to evaluate hormonal status, semen analysis and, if indicated, testicular biopsy can reveal many specific causes of infertility, some of which are reversible. Analysis of sperm morphology is now used to predict fertilizing capability in in vitro fertilization. Of these tests, semen analysis is still the most informative method available for the initial evaluation of male infertility.

Part Two
ATLAS

PLATE 1

Viable and Nonviable Spermatozoa

Figure 1 Viable and nonviable spermatozoa. Viable spermatozoon remains colorless. Nonviable spermatozoon stains eosin-red. (Eosin-nigrosin)

Figure 2 Viable and nonviable spermatozoa. Viable spermatozoon remains colorless. Nonviable spermatozoa stain eosin-red. (1% eosin Y)

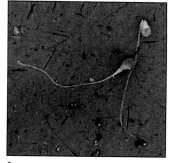

1

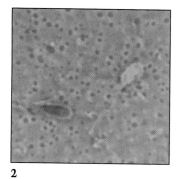

2

PLATE 2

Normal and Vacuolated Spermatozoa

Normal spermatozoa are regular in size and shape. They show ovoid heads and uncoiled, intact tailpieces. The sperm head shows 2 distinct areas, the acrosome and the postacrosomal region. The acrosome, a caplike structure, extends over the anterior two thirds of the sperm head and stains lighter than the postacrosomal region. The sperm head measures approximately 4 to 5 μm in length and 2 to 3 μm in width at the transverse line. The uncoiled tailpiece measures approximately 50 to 55 μm in length and varies in thickness from 1 μm at the midpiece to 0.1 μm at the tip.

Vacuolated spermatozoa have vacuoles that appear as holes or bubbles in the sperm head.

Figure 1   Normal spermatozoa. (Papanicolaou)

Figure 2   Normal spermatozoon. (H & E)

Figure 3   Normal spermatozoa. (Testsimplets®)

Figure 4   Vacuolated spermatozoa. (Papanicolaou)

Figure 5   Vacuolated spermatozoa. Acrosomal, nuclear, and tailpiece abnormalities. (H & E)

Figure 6   Vacuolated spermatozoa. (Testsimplets®)

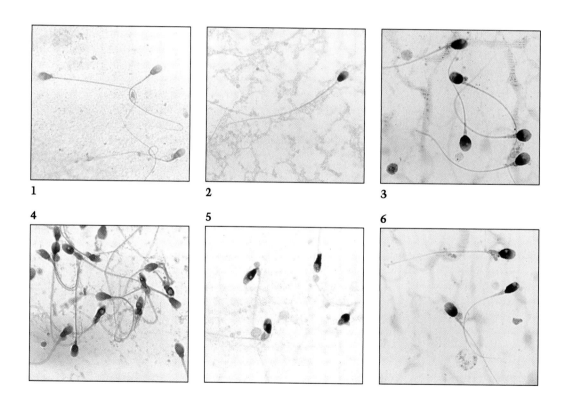

1

2

3

4

5

6

PLATE 3

Spermatozoa with Acrosomal Abnormalities

The acrosomal region may occupy less than one half of the sperm head or be missing entirely. This defect may be termed acrosomal deficiency. These spermatozoa have rounded, pointed, or flattened-off headpieces. Occasionally a spermatozoon will show enlargement or malformation of the acrosomal area.

Figure 1   Spermatozoon. Acrosomal deficiency—pointed headpiece. (Papanicolaou)

Figure 2   Spermatozoa. Acrosomal deficiency—pointed headpieces. (Papanicolaou)

Figure 3   Spermatozoa (center). Acrosomal deficiency—pointed and rounded headpieces. (Papanicolaou)

Figure 4   Spermatozoon (center). Acrosomal deficiency—flattened headpiece. (Papanicolaou)

Figure 5   Spermatozoon (center). Acrosomal deficiency—acrosome shows as small peak anterior to postacrosomal region. (Papanicolaou)

Figure 6   Spermatozoon (lower center). Enlarged and malformed acrosomal region. (Papanicolaou)

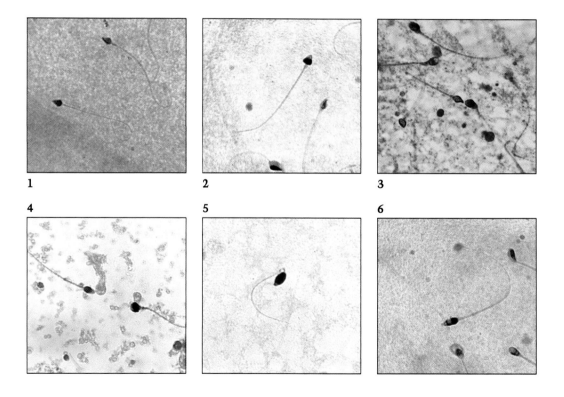

1

2

3

4

5

6

PLATE 4

Spermatozoa with Acrosomal Abnormalities

Figure 1   Two-tailed spermatozoon. Acrosomal deficiency—small rounded acrosome. (H & E)

Figure 2   Spermatozoa. Acrosomal deficiency—small rounded and pointed acrosomal regions. (H & E)

Figure 3   Spermatozoon. Acrosomal deficiency—small pointed acrosomal region. (H & E)

Figure 4   Spermatozoon (pointing right) with nuclear abnormality. Acrosomal deficiency—small pointed acrosome. Two small spermatozoa (center). Acrosomal deficiency—small pointed acrosomes. (H & E)

Figure 5   Spermatozoa. Acrosomal deficiency—small pointed acrosomes. One spermatozoon appears vacuolated. (H & E)

Figure 6   Spermatozoon (center). Malformed acrosomal region. Two spermatozoa without acrosomes. (H & E)

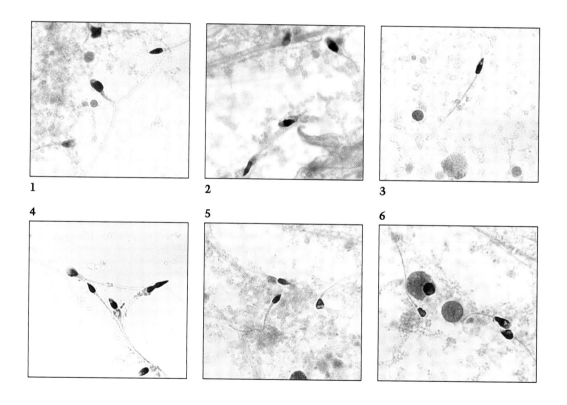

1

2

3

4

5

6

PLATE 5

Spermatozoa with Acrosomal Abnormalities

Figure 1   Spermatozoa. Acrosomal deficiency—small rounded acrosomal regions. One spermatozoon appears vacuolated. (Testsimplets®)

Figure 2   Spermatozoon. Acrosomal deficiency—small rounded acrosomal region. (Testsimplets®)

Figure 3   Spermatozoon with cytoplasmic extrusion mass. Flattened-off headpiece without acrosome. (Testsimplets®)

Figure 4   Spermatozoon with small cytoplasmic extrusion mass. Pointed headpiece without acrosome. (Testsimplets®)

Figure 5   Spermatozoon with thickened midpiece. Flattened-off headpiece with acrosomal deficiency. (Testsimplets®)

Figure 6   Two spermatozoa. Rounded headpieces without acrosomes. One spermatozoon (bottom). Acrosomal deficiency—small rounded acrosomal region. (Testsimplets®)

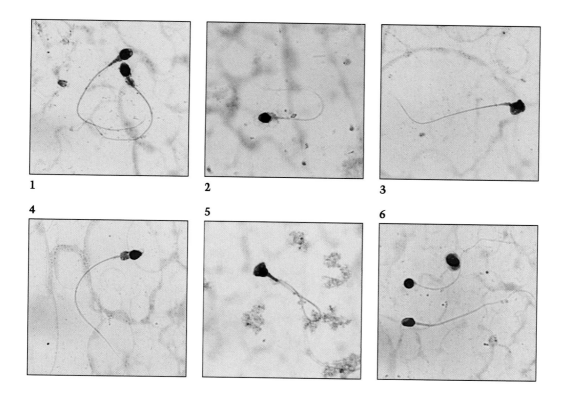

1

2

3

4

5

6

PLATE 6

Two-Headed Spermatozoa

Spermatozoa that are bicephalic or binucleate, with one tailpiece, or paired with their tailpieces intertwined, present as two-headed spermatozoa. Pairing may be caused by acrosomal deficiency, in which the spermatozoa have an affinity to pair, or by incomplete fission during spermatogenesis. Binucleate spermatozoa show two nuclei that both appear flattened on 1 side. It cannot always be determined which condition is present.

Figure 1 Spermatozoon (center). Appears to be bicephalic. (Papanicolaou)

Figure 2 Spermatozoa. Acrosomal deficiency with pairing. Two tails are clearly visible, allowing classification to be made. (Papanicolaou)

Figure 3 Spermatozoon. Acrosomal deficiency. Appears to be tricephalic with tailpieces intertwined. (Papanicolaou)

Figure 4 Spermatozoon. Appears to be binucleate. Is surrounded by cytoplasm formed during maturation. (Papanicolaou)

Figure 5 Two spermatozoa. Appear to be paired, due to incomplete fission during maturation. (Papanicolaou)

Figure 6 Three spermatozoa. Appear to be paired, due to acrosomal deficiency or to incomplete fission. (Papanicolaou)

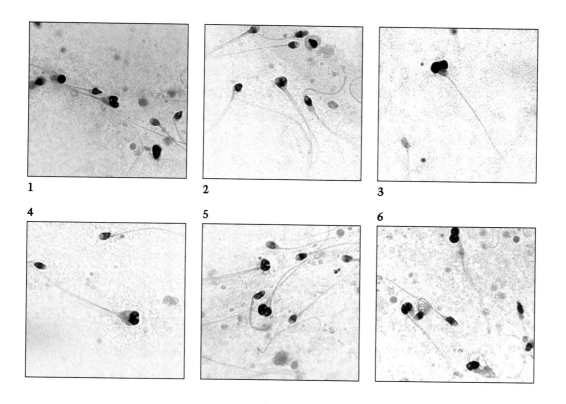

1

2

3

4

5

6

PLATE 7

Two-Headed Spermatozoa

Figure 1 Spermatozoa. Acrosomal deficiency. Appear to be bicephalic. (H & E)

Figure 2 Spermatozoa. Acrosomal deficiency. Appear to be paired or bicephalic. (H & E)

Figure 3 Spermatozoon with small cytoplasmic extrusion mass. Appears to be bicephalic. Spermine phosphate crystals are present from prolonged standing. (Testsimplets®)

Figure 4 Spermatozoa. Acrosomal deficiency. Appear to be either paired or bicephalic (or tricephalic). (Testsimplets®)

Figure 5 Spermatozoon. Appears to be binucleate and is surrounded by cytoplasm formed during maturation. (Testsimplets®)

Figure 6 Spermatozoa. Appear to be paired, due to incomplete fission during maturation. (Testsimplets®)

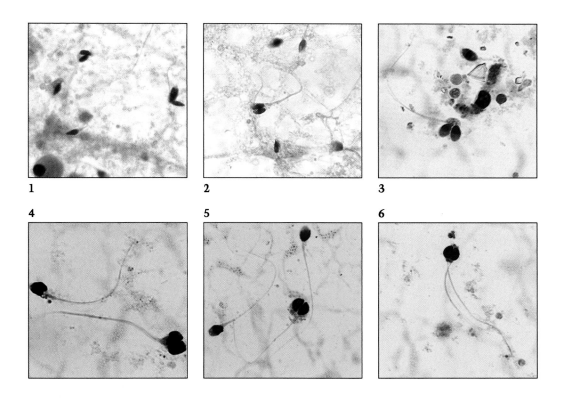

1

2

3

4

5

6

PLATE 8

Spermatozoa with Malformation of the Postacrosomal Region

Shapes may resemble bullets, mushrooms, dumbbells, and other bizarre forms. The postacrosomal cup-shaped region contains the nucleus. It may be presumed that malformation of this area demonstrates aberrations of the nucleus. Such defects may therefore be classified as nuclear abnormalities.

Figure 1 Vacuolated spermatozoon resembling an acorn. Nuclear abnormality—small flattened postacrosomal region. (Papanicolaou)

Figure 2 Spermatozoa resembling bullets and dumbbells. Nuclear abnormalities—elongated and tapered postacrosomal region. Acrosomal deficiency. (Papanicolaou)

Figure 3 Spermatozoon. Nuclear abnormality—elongated and tapered postacrosomal region, and abnormally thickened at transverse line. (Papanicolaou)

Figure 4 Spermatozoon. Nuclear abnormality—elongated postacrosomal region. (Papanicolaou)

Figure 5 Spermatozoa. Nuclear abnormalities—elongated and tapered postacrosomal region. Acrosomal deficiency. (Papanicolaou)

Figure 6 Spermatozoa resembling bullets and dumbbells. Nuclear abnormalities—elongated and tapered postacrosomal region. Acrosomal deficiency. (Papanicolaou)

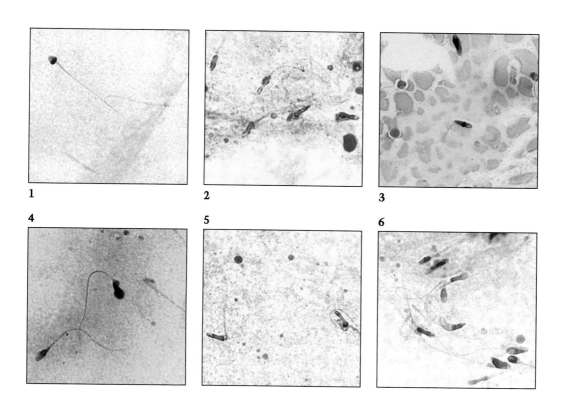

1

2

3

4

5

6

PLATE 9

Spermatozoa with Malformation of the Postacrosomal Region

Figure 1 Spermatozoon. Nuclear abnormality—elongated and tapered postacrosomal region. (H & E)

Figure 2 Spermatozoon (center). Nuclear abnormality—elongated and tapered postacrosomal region. (H & E)

Figure 3 Spermatozoon (center). Nuclear abnormality—elongated and tapered postacrosomal region. Acrosomal deficiency. (H & E)

Figure 4 Spermatozoon (center). Nuclear abnormality—elongated and tapered postacrosomal region. (H & E)

Figure 5 Megalospermatozoon (center). Nuclear abnormality—elongated postacrosomal region. (H & E)

Figure 6 Spermatozoon resembling a mushroom (lower center). Nuclear abnormality—elongated and tapered postacrosomal region. (H & E)

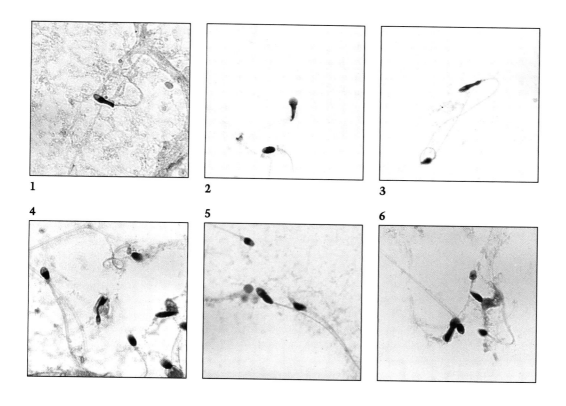

PLATE   10

Spermatozoa with Malformation of the Postacrosomal Region

Figure 1   Spermatozoon resembling a dumbbell. Nuclear abnormality—elongated and tapered postacrosomal region. (Testsimplets®)

Figure 2   Spermatozoon (lower center). Nuclear abnormality—elongated and tapered postacrosomal region. (Testsimplets®)

Figure 3   Spermatozoon (center). Nuclear abnormality—elongated and tapered postacrosomal region. (Testsimplets®)

Figure 4   Spermatozoon (left center) resembling a mushroom. Nuclear abnormality—elongated and tapered postacrosomal region. Other spermatozoa. Acrosomal deficiency. (Testsimplets®)

Figure 5   Spermatozoon (lower center). Nuclear abnormality—elongated and tapered postacrosomal region. Acrosome absent. (Testsimplets®)

Figure 6   Spermatozoon. Nuclear abnormality—narrowed postacrosomal region. Acrosomal abnormality. (Testsimplets®)

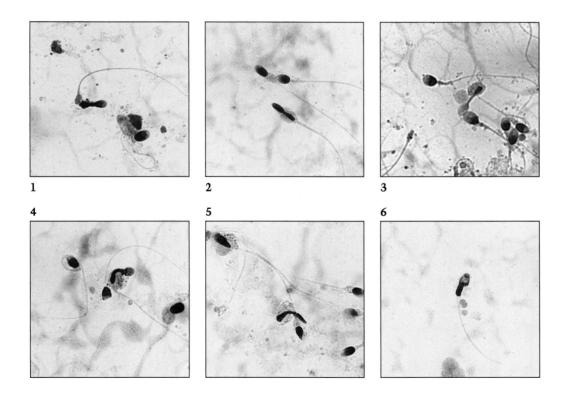

1

2

3

4

5

6

PLATE 11

Spermatozoa with Malformation of the Postacrosomal Region

Figure 1 Spermatozoon (left). Nuclear abnormality—elongated postacrosomal region. Acrosome absent. Spermatozoa (upper right). Kinked midpieces and coiled tailpieces. (Testsimplets®)

Figure 2 Spermatozoa. Nuclear abnormalities—elongated postacrosomal region. Acrosomal deficiency. (Papanicolaou)

Figure 3 Spermatozoon. Nuclear abnormality—small flattened postacrosomal region. Acrosome absent. (Papanicolaou)

Figure 4 Spermatozoon (center). Nuclear abnormality—small protuberance anterior to postacrosomal region. Acrosome absent. (Papanicolaou)

Figure 5 Spermatozoon (center). Nuclear abnormality—enlarged irregular postacrosomal region. Acrosome absent. (Papanicolaou)

Figure 6 Spermatozoon (center). Nuclear abnormality—enlarged irregular postacrosomal region. Acrosome absent. (Papanicolaou)

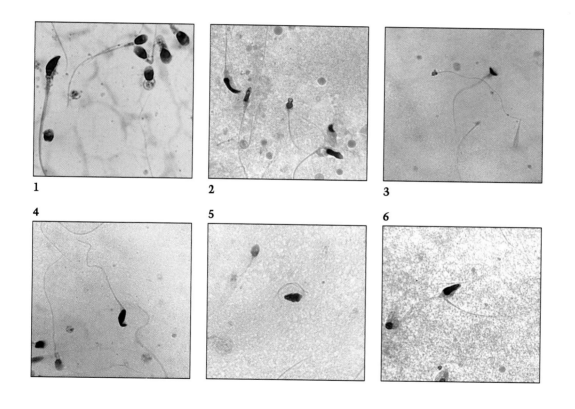

1

2

3

4

5

6

PLATE 12

Variation of Size of Spermatozoa

Sperm heads that vary greatly in dimensions from 4 to 5 μm in length and 2 to 3 μm in width at the transverse line are classified as megalospermatozoa (macrospermatozoa) if abnormally large or microspermatozoa if abnormally small.

Figure 1   Megalospermatozoon. Coiled tailpiece. Microspermatozoon (lower right). (Papanicolaou)

Figure 2   Megalospermatozoon. Slightly thickened midpiece region. (Papanicolaou)

Figure 3   Megalospermatozoon (upper center). Nuclear and acrosomal abnormalities. (H & E)

Figure 4   Megalospermatozoon. Shortened tailpiece. (H & E)

Figure 5   Megalospermatozoon. Absence of acrosome. (Testsimplets®)

Figure 6   Megalospermatozoon (left center). Microspermatozoon (right of megalospermatozoon). Absence of acrosome. (Testsimplets®)

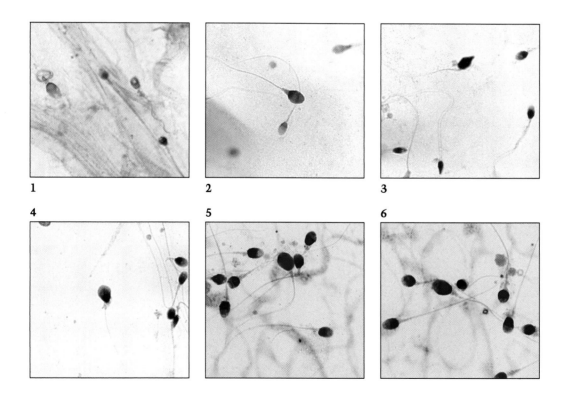

1

2

3

4

5

6

PLATE 13

Variation of Size of Spermatozoa

Figure 1   Three microspermatozoa. Acrosomal deficiency. (Papanicolaou)

Figure 2   Microspermatozoon (center). Acrosomal deficiency. (Papanicolaou)

Figure 3   Microspermatozoon (center). Absence of acrosome. (H & E)

Figure 4   Microspermatozoon (center). Contrast with normal size spermatozoa around it. (H & E)

Figure 5   Microspermatozoon (far right). (Testsimplets®)

Figure 6   Microspermatozoon. Nuclear abnormality and absence of acrosome. (Testsimplets®)

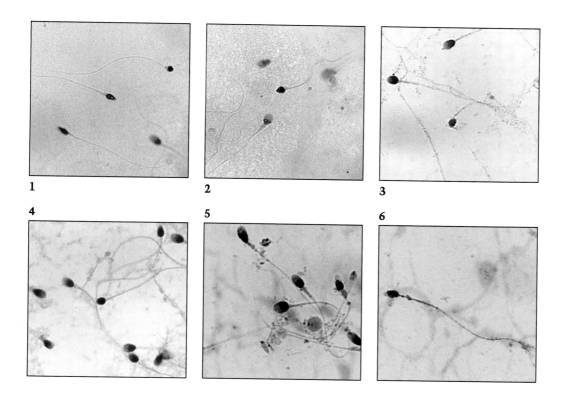

1

2

3

4

5

6

PLATE 14

Variation of Size of Spermatozoa

Figure 1 Spermatozoa. Size variation. Nuclear and acrosomal abnormalities. (Testsimplets®)

Figure 2 Microspermatozoon and megalospermatozoon. (Testsimplets®)

Figure 3 Spermatozoa. Size variation. Acrosomal deficiency. (Testsimplets®)

Figure 4 Spermatozoa. Size variation. Microspermatozoon (lower center). Nuclear abnormality, absence of acrosome, and shortened tailpiece. (Papanicolaou)

Figure 5 Spermatozoa. Size variation. Tailpiece abnormalities. (Papanicolaou)

Figure 6 Spermatozoa. Size variation. (Papanicolaou)

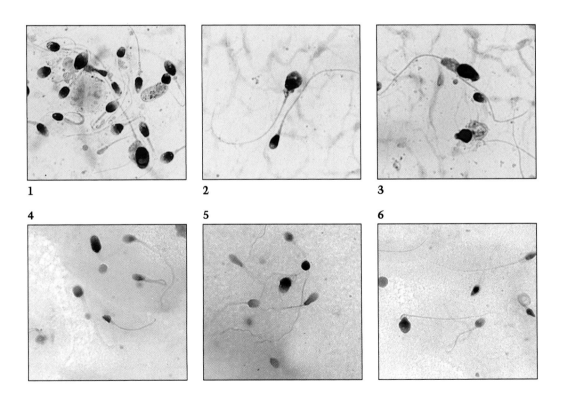

1   2   3

4   5   6

PLATE 15

Spermatozoa with Variation in Length of the Tailpiece

Tailpieces may be considerably shorter or longer than 55 μm.

Figure 1   Vacuolated spermatozoon. Shortened tailpiece. (Papanicolaou)

Figure 2   Spermatozoon (right). Shortened tailpiece. Spermatozoon (center). Curled tailpiece. (H & E)

Figure 3   Spermatozoon. Shortened tailpiece. Acrosomal deficiency. (H & E)

Figure 4   Spermatozoon. Shortened tailpiece. Acrosomal deficiency. (Testsimplets®)

Figure 5   Vacuolated spermatozoon. Shortened tailpiece. (Testsimplets®)

Figure 6   Spermatozoon (upper right). Lengthened tailpiece. (H & E)

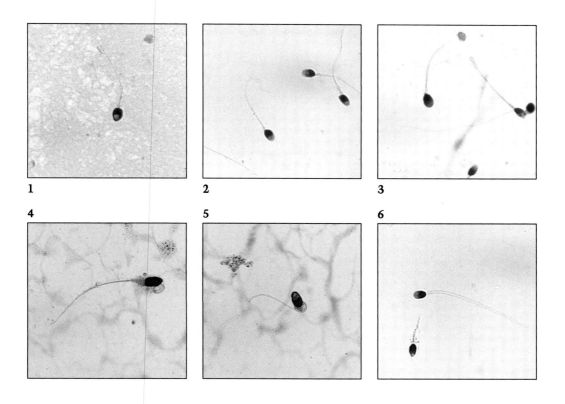

1

2

3

4

5

6

PLATE 16

Spermatozoa with Lengthened Neckpiece

The neckpiece of the normal spermatozoon is barely discernible by light microscopy. Spermatozoa that show lengthened neckpieces display a lengthened axial filament at the base of the headpiece. This filament usually bends, causing the headpiece to fall backward on the midpiece at a 90° angle or greater.

Figure 1 Two spermatozoa. Lengthened neckpieces with headpieces bent backward. (Papanicolaou)

Figure 2 Immature spermatozoon. Lengthened neckpiece. (Papanicolaou)

Figure 3 Spermatozoon (center). Lengthened neckpiece with headpiece bent backward. (H & E)

Figure 4 Spermatozoon. Lengthened neckpiece. Polymorphonuclear white blood cells. (H & E)

Figure 5 Spermatozoa. Lengthened neckpieces with headpieces bent backward. Coiled tailpiece. Nuclear and acrosomal abnormalities. (Testsimplets®)

Figure 6 Spermatozoon. Lengthened neckpiece. Bizarre headpiece with nuclear and acrosomal abnormalities. (Testsimplets®)

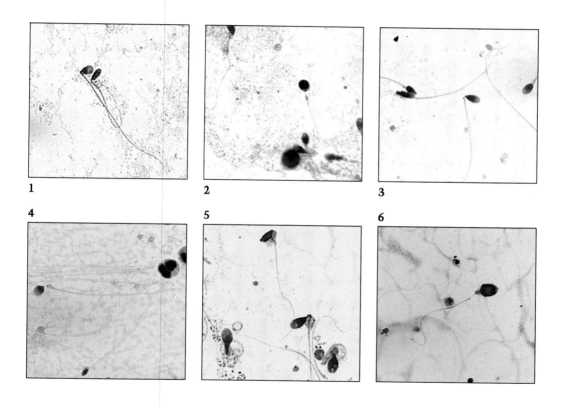

1

2

3

4

5

6

PLATE 17

Spermatozoa with Coiled Tailpiece

The tailpiece may curl below the headpiece or encircle the entire spermatozoon.

Figure 1 Spermatozoa. Coiled tailpiece. Acrosomal deficiency. (Papanicolaou)

Figure 2 Spermatozoa. Coiled tailpiece. Acrosomal deficiency. (H & E)

Figure 3 Spermatozoa. Coiled tailpiece. Acrosomal deficiency. (H & E)

Figure 4 Spermatozoa. Curled tailpiece. Acrosomal deficiency. (Testsimplets®)

Figure 5 Spermatozoa. Curled and coiled tailpieces. Acrosomal deficiency. (Testsimplets®)

Figure 6 Spermatozoa. Coiled tailpieces. Cytoplasmic extrusion masses on coiled tailpieces. (Testsimplets®)

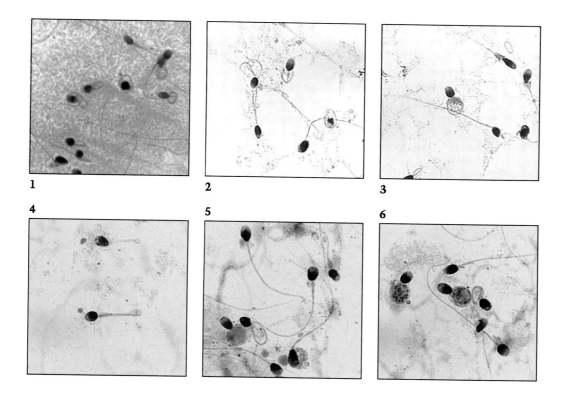

1

2

3

4

5

6

PLATE 18

Spermatozoa with Midpiece Abnormality

The tailpiece may be thickened or kinked in the midpiece region.

Figure 1 Spermatozoa. Thickened midpiece. Cytoplasmic extrusion masses and acrosomal deficiency. Vacuolation. (Papanicolaou)

Figure 2 Spermatozoa. Kinked midpiece (left). Coiled tailpiece (right). (Papanicolaou)

Figure 3 Two spermatozoa without acrosomes. Pairing in midpiece region. (Papanicolaou)

Figure 4 Spermatozoon. Thickened midpiece region. (H & E)

Figure 5 Two spermatozoa. Kinked and thickened midpiece region. (Testsimplets®)

Figure 6 Spermatozoon. Thickened midpiece region. (Testsimplets®)

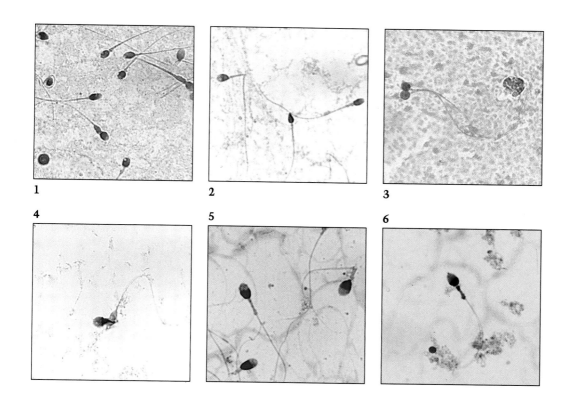

1

2

3

4

5

6

PLATE 19

Multitailed Spermatozoa

Two or more tailpieces may arise from the base of the headpiece or from the annulus of the midpiece region.

Figure 1 Multitailed spermatozoon without acrosome. Two tailpieces arise from base of headpiece. Acrosomal deficiency. (Papanicolaou)

Figure 2 Multitailed spermatozoon without acrosome. Two tailpieces arise from disorganized midpiece. (Papanicolaou)

Figure 3 Multitailed spermatozoon. Acrosomal deficiency. Two tailpieces arise from midpiece. Other spermatozoa. Nuclear and acrosomal abnormalities. (Papanicolaou)

Figure 4 Multitailed spermatozoon. Acrosomal and nuclear abnormalities. Two tailpieces arise from midpiece. (H & E)

Figure 5 Megalospermatozoon. Two tailpieces arise from disorganized midpiece. (Testsimplets®)

Figure 6 Megalospermatozoon. Two tailpieces arise from base of headpiece. (Testsimplets®)

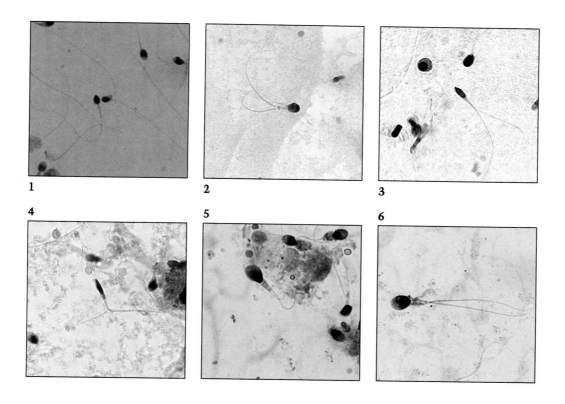

1

2

3

4

5

6

PLATE 20

Spermatozoa with Cytoplasmic Extrusion Mass

Excess cytoplasmic material formed during maturation may be present in the midpiece region.

Figure 1 Spermatozoon (upper center). Acrosomal deficiency. Cytoplasmic extrusion mass stained bright pink. (Papanicolaou)

Figure 2 Spermatozoon. Cytoplasmic extrusion mass stained blue. (Papanicolaou)

Figure 3 Spermatozoon (center). Cytoplasmic extrusion mass. Shortened tailpiece. (H & E)

Figure 4 Spermatozoon (upper center). Cytoplasmic extrusion mass. Spermatozoon (lower center). Kinked midpiece. (H & E)

Figure 5 Spermatozoa. Cytoplasmic extrusion mass. (Testsimplets®)

Figure 6 Spermatozoon. Coiled tailpiece with cytoplasmic extrusion mass. Two-tailed spermatozoon. (Testsimplets®)

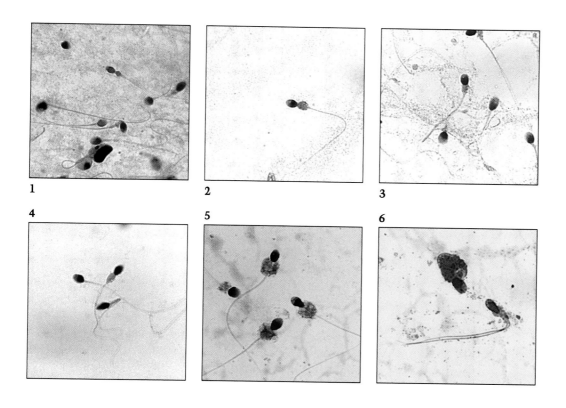

PLATE 21

Immature Spermatozoa and Polymorphonuclear White Blood Cells

Immature spermatozoa present as cells with residual bodies and nuclei that are not interconnected. The nuclear:cytoplasmic ratio of the developing germ cell varies greatly. Precise classification of the maturing germ cells into categories of primary spermatocyte, secondary spermatocyte, and spermatid is difficult and unnecessary during routine semen analysis. It is therefore beyond the scope of this book. It is, however, important to distinguish these cells from polymorphonuclear white blood cells. In contrast to the variations of the germ cell, polymorphonuclear leukocytes are relatively regular in size and shape. Their nuclei are characterized by 3 or more interconnected lobes and a consistent nuclear:cytoplasmic ratio. Late stage spermatids can be identified by the presence of a tailpiece.

Figure 1   Polymorphonuclear white blood cells. Regular size and shape, consistent nuclear:cytoplasmic ratio, and nuclei with interconnected lobes. (Papanicolaou)

Figure 2   Two polymorphonuclear white blood cells. Regular size and shape, consistent nuclear:cytoplasmic ratio, and nuclei with interconnected lobes. Bacteria. (Papanicolaou)

Figure 3   Polymorphonuclear white blood cells. Regular size and shape, consistent nuclear:cytoplasmic ratio, and nuclei with interconnected lobes. Spermatozoon. Coiled tailpiece. (H & E)

Figure 4   Polymorphonuclear white blood cells. Regular size and shape, consistent nuclear:cytoplasmic ratio, and nuclei with interconnected lobes. Spermatozoa. Lengthened neckpiece. (H & E)

Figure 5   Polymorphonuclear white blood cell. Nuclei with interconnected lobes. (Testsimplets®)

Figure 6   Polymorphonuclear white blood cells. Regular size and shape, consistent nuclear:cytoplasmic ratio, and nuclei with interconnected lobes. (Testsimplets®)

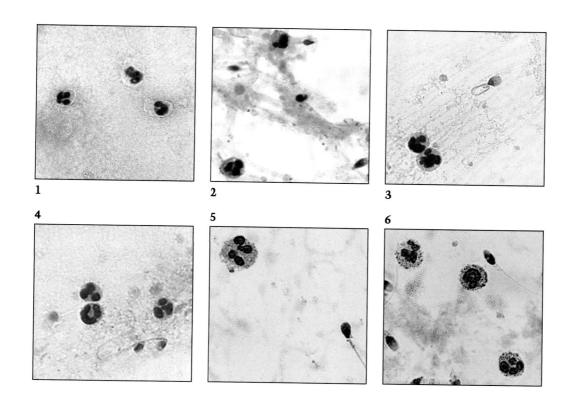

1

2

3

4

5

6

PLATE 22

Immature Spermatozoa and Polymorphonuclear White Blood Cells

Figure 1   Maturing germ cells. Size variation. Nuclei not interconnected. (Papanicolaou)

Figure 2   Maturing germ cells. Size variation. Spermatid (right center) with tailpiece. Germ cell (center). Pear shape distinctive to developing germ cell. (Papanicolaou)

Figure 3   Maturing germ cells. Size variation. Nuclei not interconnected. Germ cell (far left). Pear shape distinctive to developing germ cell. (Papanicolaou)

Figure 4   Maturing germ cells. Size variation. Nuclei not interconnected. (Papanicolaou)

Figure 5   Maturing germ cell. Eccentric nuclei with low nuclear:cytoplasmic ratio. (Papanicolaou)

Figure 6   Maturing germ cells. Nuclear variation but little variation in size and shape. Germ cell (lower center). Pear shape distinctive to developing germ cell. (Papanicolaou)

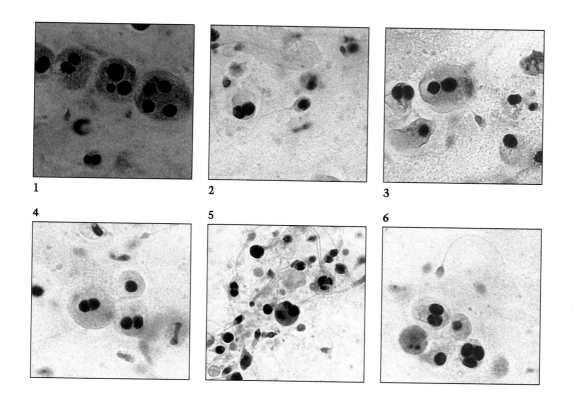

1

2

3

4

5

6

PLATE 23

Immature Spermatozoa and Polymorphonuclear White Blood Cells

Figure 1 Spermatid with tailpiece. (H & E)

Figure 2 Maturing germ cells. Germ cell (upper center). Pear shape distinctive to developing germ cell. (H & E)

Figure 3 Maturing germ cells. Size variation. Nuclei not interconnected. (H & E).

Figure 4 Maturing germ cells. Size variation. Nuclei not interconnected. (H & E).

Figure 5 Maturing germ cells. Size variation. Nuclei not interconnected. (H & E).

Figure 6 Maturing germ cell. Eccentric nuclei with low nuclear:cytoplasmic ratio. (H & E)

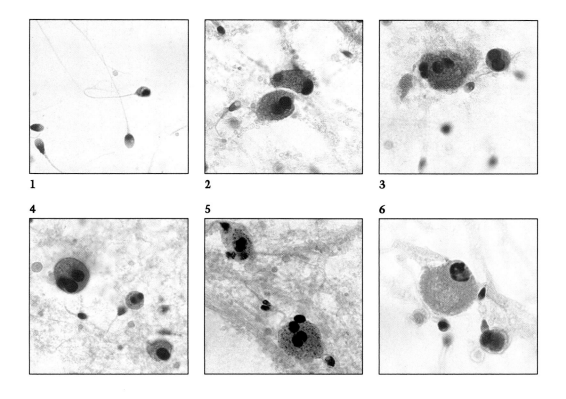

PLATE 24

Immature Spermatozoa and Polymorphonuclear White Blood Cells

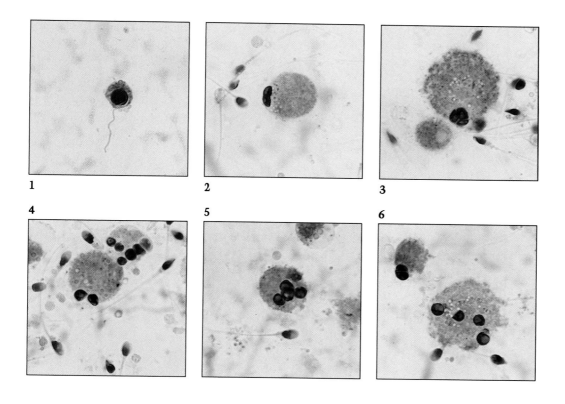

PLATE 25

Presence of Bacteria and Spermine Phosphate Crystals

Bacteria may be present in seminal fluid due to prolonged standing or to an inflammatory process of the male reproductive tract. Polymorphonuclear white blood cells, frequently accompanied by agglutination of the spermatozoa and/ or the semen, are indicative of an inflammatory process.

Spermine phosphate crystals form in semen upon prolonged standing. They are, therefore, more commonly found on the Testsimplets® slide, because it is a wet mount and may be subject to prolonged standing prior to being read.

Figure 1   Spermatozoa. Bacteria. Polymorphonuclear white blood cell. (Papanicolaou)

Figure 2   Spermatozoa. Bacteria. Agglutination of spermatozoa. (H & E)

Figure 3   Spermatozoa. Bacteria. (Testsimplets®)

Figure 4   Spermatozoa. Spermine phosphate crystals. (Testsimplets®)

Figure 5   Maturing germ cells. Spermine phosphate crystals. (Testsimplets®)

Figure 6   Maturing germ cells. Spermine phosphate crystals. (Testsimplets®)

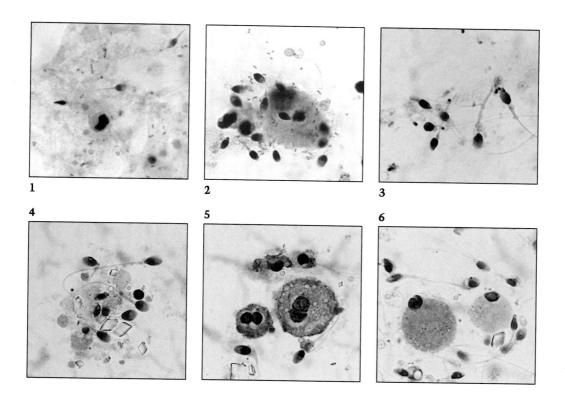

1

2

3

4

5

6

PLATE 26

Histologic Sections of the Male Reproductive Tract

Figure 1 Normal seminiferous tubules in 47-year-old male. (40×, H & E)

Figure 2 Normal spermatogenesis. Mature spermatozoa in larger tubule and Leydig cells in interstitium. (100×, H & E)

Figure 3 Seminiferous tubules lined only by Sertoli cells in germ cell aplasia. (100×, H & E)

Figure 4 Sloughing of immature spermatocytes in tubular lumen. (250×, H & E)

Figure 5 Maturation arrest with absence of mature spermatozoa. (250×, H & E)

Figure 6 Ducts of epididymis filled with spermatozoa. (100×, H & E)

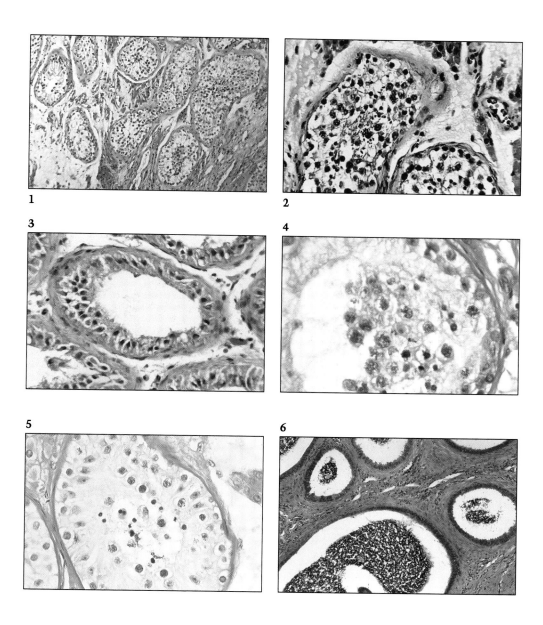

1

2

3

4

5

6

Part Three

PROCEDURES

CHAPTER 6

Laboratory Techniques

Safety Precautions for Handling Semen Specimens

Infectious agents such as the human immunodeficiency virus (HIV) and hepatitis B virus may be transmitted through semen. Therefore, safety precautions generally taken when handling any body fluid must also be followed when handling semen specimens. The following recommendations are advised.

1. All specimens should be treated as infectious.
2. Specimens should be transported in closed plastic bags with requisitions attached to the outside of the bag.
3. Protective gloves should be worn.
4. Protective clothing such as lab coats or aprons should be worn.
5. Nothing should be pipetted by mouth.
6. No eating, drinking, or smoking should be allowed in the work area.
7. Countertops should be disinfected after spills and when work is completed with 1% sodium hypochlorite or 70% alcohol.
8. Contaminated materials should be discarded in "biohazard bags."
9. Closed "biohazard bags" should be autoclaved prior to disposal.

1.1 Guaiac Test for Blood

Reagents

1. Glacial acetic acid
2. Gum guaiac

3. 95% ethyl alcohol

4. 3% hydrogen peroxide

Prepared Reagents

1. Gum guaiac solution (must be prepared fresh every 30 days)
   a. Add 120 mL 95% ethyl alcohol to 2 g gum guaiac.
   b. Swirl gently to mix.
   c. Allow to stand until dissolved at room temperature.
   d. Store in a dark bottle.

Procedure

1. Place 3 to 5 drops of semen in white dish.
2. Add 3 drops of glacial acetic acid (to release hemoglobin from intact red blood cells).
3. Add 3 drops of gum guaiac solution.
4. Add 3 drops of 3% hydrogen peroxide.
5. Observe for 1 minute. Development of green or blue color indicates positive reaction.

1.2 Liquefying Viscous Semen in 5% Alpha Amylase in Locke's Solution

Reagents

1. Sodium chloride
2. Calcium chloride
3. Potassium chloride
4. Sodium bicarbonate
5. Glucose
6. Alpha amylase from human saliva (Sigma)

Prepared Reagents

1. Locke's solution
   a. Place 9.00 g of sodium chloride into 1 liter volumetric flask.
   b. Add 0.24 g of calcium chloride.

  c. Add 0.42 g of potassium chloride.

  d. Add 0.10 g of sodium bicarbonate.

  e. Add 1.00 g of glucose.

  f. Add enough distilled water to make 1 liter.

  g. Shake well to mix.

2. 5% alpha amylase

  a. Prepare 5% solution of alpha amylase in Locke's solution.

Procedure

1. Mix equal volumes of semen and 5% alpha amylase in test tube.
2. Allow to stand until semen liquefies. (A larger amount of alpha amylase may be added if necessary.)
3. Multiply sperm count by factor to compensate for this initial dilution of semen (eg, if equal volumes of semen and alpha amylase were used, multiply sperm count by 2).
4. No compensation is necessary for motility ratings.

1.3 Sperm Count (Sperm Density)

Procedure

1. Allow specimen to liquefy.
2. Agitate by swirling container gently for 30 seconds to permit fractions of semen to mix well.
3. Make 1:20 dilution of seminal fluid in water. To do this, draw semen to 0.5 mark and water to 11 mark of white blood cell pipet.*
4. Mix on mechanical blood pipet shaker or shake by hand for 2 to 3 minutes.
5. Discard 3 drops from pipet.
6. Load into counting chamber (standard Neubauer hemocytometer).
7. Allow to settle for 2 to 3 minutes.
8. Survey counting chamber under 40✕ magnification using light microscope to determine counting area. (See Sperm Density, p. 7.)
9. Count spermatozoa.
10. Calculate number of spermatozoa per mL. (See Sperm Density, p. 7 for formula and counting/dilution options.)

* Dilutions of 1:10 or smaller can be made if very few spermatozoa are present. Semen can be diluted in a test tube using micropipets if desired. Water is the

preferred diluent because it immobilizes the spermatozoa, is readily available, and requires no preparation.

1.4 Sperm Motility

Materials

1. Petroleum jelly

Procedure

1. Rim large coverslip with petroleum jelly.
2. Place 1 drop of liquefied semen on labeled glass slide.
3. Place petroleum jelly–rimmed coverslip over drop.
4. Exert gentle pressure on coverslip with end of pencil or other blunt instrument to spread drop evenly.
5. Either leave slide at room temperature or incubate at 37 °C in a hot air incubator. (Note: 37 °C closely approximates the temperature of the female reproductive tract, but results in a faster decline of motility than slides incubated at 23 °C to 25 °C. If room temperature falls below 22 °C, motility also declines faster. Therefore, it is recommended that slides be incubated at room temperature, unless room temperature is extremely erratic. In these instances, incubation at 37 °C will give consistent results, albeit slightly lower rates in general.)
6. Examine slide under $40\times$ magnification using light microscope.
7. Determine percentage of motile spermatozoa. (See Sperm Motility, p. 10, if motility is not evenly distributed.)
8. Determine quality of motility using rating scale of $1+$ to $4+$. (See Sperm Motility, p. 10.)
9. Evaluate motility immediately upon preparation of the motility slide and once every 60 minutes for 6 hours after preparation.
10. Note and report agglutination of spermatozoa, WBCs, RBCs, crystals, and other debris.

1.5 Swim-Up Test

Reagents

1. Penicillin G(K)
2. Ca lactate, 4.5 H_2O, 1mM

3. $NaHCO_3$, 20mM
4. $KHCO_3$, 5mM
5. $MgSO_4 \cdot 7H_2O$, 1mM
6. Ham's F-10 nutrient media powder with glutamine, without sodium bicarbonate (Sigma Chemical Company)
7. Distilled water HPLC grade

Prepared Reagents

1. Ham's nutrient media
    a. Dissolve 4.900 g Ham's F-10 nutrient media powder in 482 mL distilled water.
    b. Add 0.025 g penicillin G(K).
    c. Add 0.062 g $MgSO_4$.
    d. Add 0.150 g Ca lactate with vigorous mixing.
    e. Dissolve 0.840 g $NaHCO_3$ and 0.254 g $KHCO_3$ in 10 mL distilled water. Add to Ham's solution. Mix.
    f. Adjust osmolarity to 280 mosm.
    g. Adjust pH to 7.3 to 7.5.
    h. Filter through Nalgene filter unit.
    i. Store at 3 °C to 8 °C in sterile test tubes.

Procedure

1. Place 1 mL of semen into 15 mL conical tube.
2. Add 3 mL warmed (37 °C) Ham's nutrient media. Mix. Centrifuge at 1100 rpm at 20 °C for 10 minutes.
3. Remove supernatant with transfer pipet.
4. Add 2 mL warmed (37 °C) Ham's nutrient media to pellet. Mix. Transfer to 12 × 75 mm plastic test tube.
5. Centrifuge at 1100 rpm at 20 °C for 10 minutes.
6. Remove 1.9 mL of supernatant with micropipet.
7. Overlay pellet with 1 mL warmed (37 °C) Ham's nutrient media, taking care not to disturb the pellet.
8. Place in 37 °C, 5% CO_2 incubator for 1 hour.
9. Remove top 800 μL (0.8 mL) of fluid with transfer pipet. Place in 12 × 75 mm test tube.
10. Load standard Neubauer hemocytometer with drop of fluid from 12 × 75 mm test tube in step 9.

11. Count spermatozoa seen in all 25 secondary squares of primary square E. (See p. 7 for explanation of hemocytometer squares.)
12. Calculate the number of spermatozoa that completed the swim-up using the formula:

swim-up spermatozoa/mL = Number of spermatozoa counted $\times 10^4$.

1.6 Cervical Mucus Penetration (Penetrak® Test)*

Materials

1. Flat capillary tubes filled with estrous bovine cervical mucus (supplied with kit). (Store at -12 °C to -20 °C in original container.)

Procedure

1. Thaw 2 capillary tubes at room temperature (20 °C to 25 °C) in an upright position with score marks at upper end.
2. Swirl freshly liquefied semen to mix.
3. Pipet 200 μL (0.2 mL) semen into sample cup with conical bottom.
4. Break capillary tubes at score mark. Discard short end of tube.
5. Place open ends of capillary tubes into sample cup.
6. Incubate at room temperature for 90 minutes.
7. Remove 1 capillary tube from sample cup. Wipe off excess semen.
8. Place capillary tube on ruled microscope slide (supplied with kit).
9. Examine capillary tube using light microscope for spermatozoa.
10. Determine the spermatozoon that has traveled furthest into tube.
11. Record this distance using scale printed on ruled microscope slide.
12. Repeat steps 7–11 using second capillary tube.
13. Average results of 2 readings.
14. Normal penetration is greater than or equal to 30 mm.

*Specimen should be evaluated within 3 hours of collection.

1.7 Viability Stain—1% Eosin Y Solution

Reagents

1. Isotonic phosphate buffer
2. Eosin Y

Prepared Reagents

1. 1% eosin Y solution
   a. Prepare a 1% (w/v) eosin Y solution in isotonic phosphate buffer with pH 7.5.

Procedure

1. Place 1 to 2 drops of semen in test tube.
2. Add equal volume of 1% eosin Y solution.
3. Allow to stand for 2 minutes.
4. Place 5μL (0.005 mL) of eosin-semen mixture on labeled glass slide.
5. Smear drop to feather edge (similar to edge made in preparing blood smear).
6. Allow smear to dry.
7. Do not coverslip.
8. Examine smear under 40× or greater magnification using light microscope.
9. Determine percentage of spermatozoa that remain colorless. (Nonviable spermatozoa stain eosin-red. Viable spermatozoa remain colorless.)

1.8 Viability Stain—Eosin-Nigrosin Solutions

Reagents

1. Eosin Y
2. Nigrosin

Prepared Reagents

1. 1% eosin Y solution
   a. Prepare 1% (w/v) eosin Y solution in distilled water.
2. 10% nigrosin solution
   a. Prepare 10% (w/v) nigrosin solution in distilled water.

Procedure

1. Place 1 to 2 drops of semen in test tube.
2. Add 2 drops of 1% eosin Y solution.
3. Allow to stand at room temperature for 30 seconds.
4. Add 3 drops of 10% nigrosin solution.

5. Immediately place 5 μL (0.005 mL) of eosin-nigrosin-semen mixture on labeled glass slide.

6. Smear drop to feather edge (as in preparation of blood smear).

7. Allow smear to dry.

8. Coverslip.

9. Examine smear under 40$\times$ or greater magnification using light microscope.

10. Determine percentage of spermatozoa that remain colorless. (Nonviable spermatozoa stain eosin-red. Viable spermatozoa remain colorless.)

1.9 Testsimplets® Technique for Sperm Analysis (Boehringer Mannheim)

Background

Testsimplets® ready-for-use microscope slides are prestained with N-methylene blue and cresyl violet acetate. They provide a fast, reliable, and convenient method for cytological study of seminal fluid, negating need for extensive staining equipment.

Materials

1. Testsimplets®

Procedure

1. Allow semen to liquefy at room temperature.

2. Using a pipet, bacteriology loop, or other dropping device, apply 5 μL (0.005 mL) of semen directly to center of stained portion of labeled Testsimplets® slide.

3. Place provided coverslip on drop of semen.

4. Gently press center of coverslip with pencil to spread semen into very thin layer.*

5. Slide may be sealed with nail polish if desired.

6. Allow slide to stand at least 30 minutes at room temperature.

7. Slide is ideally read within 24 hours under oil immersion magnification. Slide will remain stable for at least 24 hours when refrigerated at 8 °C.

*Preparation of a thin smear is essential. Semen need not completely cover stained area. Thick preparations result in incomplete immobilization of spermatozoa and excessive movement of seminal fluid, making interpretation under oil immersion difficult.

1.10 Slide Preparation for Stains (Papanicolaou; Hematoxylin and Eosin)

Materials

1. Spray-Cyte® (Clay Adams)*
2. Glass slides

Procedure

1. Allow semen to liquefy at room temperature.
2. Place 1 drop of semen at 1 end of labeled glass slide.
3. Place second slide on top of drop.
4. Pull second slide across bottom slide, smearing semen entire length of slide.
5. Spray resultant smear immediately with Spray-Cyte®.
6. Dry at room temperature.

*If Spray-Cyte® is not available, the smear may be air dried and fixed in a solution of equal parts of 95% ethyl alcohol and ether for 5 to 15 minutes. (WHO)

1.11 Papanicolaou Stain

Reagents

1. Light green SF yellow, C.I. No. 42095
2. Ethyl alcohol
3. Bismarck brown, C.I. NO. 21000
4. Eosin
5. Phosphotungstic acid
6. Orange G, C.I. No. 16230
7. Hematoxylin, C.I. 75290
8. Aluminum ammonium sulfate (alum)
9. Mercuric oxide
10. Hydrochloric acid
11. Xylene
12. Permount

Prepared Reagents

1. Eosin-alcohol (EA-65) stain
   a. Solution A (0.1% light green)

1. Place 50 mL 2% light green SF yellow, C.I. No. 42095, in dark glass bottle.
   2. Add 950 mL 95% ethyl alcohol.
   b. Solution B (0.5% bismarck brown)
      1. Place 5 mL 10% bismarck brown, C.I. No. 21000, in dark glass bottle.
      2. Add 95 mL 95% ethyl alcohol.
   c. Solution C (0.5% eosin)
      1. Place 5 g eosin in dark glass bottle.
      2. Add 1000 mL 95% ethyl alcohol.
   d. Mix the following in dark glass bottle.
      1. 225 mL solution A
      2. 100 mL solution B
      3. 6 g phosphotungstic acid
      4. 450 mL solution C
      5. 225 mL ethyl alcohol
2. Orange-G (OG-6) stain
   a. Place 50 mL 10% orange G, C.I. No. 16230, in dark glass bottle.
   b. Add 950 mL ethyl alcohol.
   c. Add 0.15 g phosphotungstic acid.
   d. Mix.
3. Harris' hematoxylin
   a. Solution A
      1. Place 5 g hematoxylin, C.I. 75290, in glass bottle.
      2. Add 50 mL absolute ethyl alcohol.
      3. Dissolve hematoxylin in alcohol.
   b. Solution B
      1. Place 100 g aluminum ammonium sulfate (alum) in glass bottle.
      2. Add 1000 mL distilled water.
      3. Dissolve alum in water with aid of heat. Bring to boil.
   c. While solution B is boiling, add solution A and bring to boil again.
   d. Remove from heat.
   e. Immediately add 2.5 g mercuric oxide.
   f. Stir solution until dark purple color appears.
   g. Plunge flask into water bath to cool.
   h. Filter and store in dark bottle.

4. 95% ethyl alcohol
   a. Prepare 95% solution of ethyl alcohol in distilled water.
5. 80% ethyl alcohol
   a. Prepare 80% solution of ethyl alcohol in distilled water.
6. 70% ethyl alcohol
   a. Prepare 70% solution of ethyl alcohol in distilled water.
7. 50% ethyl alcohol
   a. Prepare 50% solution of ethyl alcohol in distilled water.
8. 0.25% hydrochloric acid
   a. Prepare 0.25% solution of hydrochloric acid in distilled water.

Procedure

1. Hydration
   a. 80% ethyl alcohol, 10 dips
   b. 70% ethyl alcohol, 10 dips
   c. 50% ethyl alcohol, 10 dips
   d. Water, 10 dips
2. Nuclear stain
   a. Place in half strength Harris' hematoxylin for 6 minutes.
3. Rinse
   a. Water, 10 dips
   b. Water, 10 dips
4. Differentiation
   a. 0.25% HCl, 6 dips
5. Bluing
   a. Place in running tap water for 6 minutes.
6. Dehydration
   a. 50% ethyl alcohol, 10 dips
   b. 70% ethyl alcohol, 10 dips
   c. 80% ethyl alcohol, 10 dips
   d. 95% ethyl alcohol, 10 dips
7. Cytoplasmic stain
   a. Place in OG-6 for 1½ minutes.
8. Rinse

    a. 95% ethyl alcohol, 10 dips

    b. 95% ethyl alcohol, 10 dips

    c. 95% ethyl alcohol, 10 dips

9. Cytoplasmic stain

    a. Place in EA-65 for 1½ minutes.

10. Rinse

    a. 95% ethyl alcohol, 10 dips

    b. 95% ethyl alcohol, 10 dips

    c. 95% ethyl alcohol, 10 dips

11. Dehydration

    a. 100% ethyl alcohol, 10 dips

    b. 100% ethyl alcohol, 10 dips

    c. 100% ethyl alcohol, 10 dips

12. Clearing

    a. Xylene, 10 dips

    b. Xylene, 10 dips

    c. Xylene, 10 dips

13. Mount

    a. Place 1 drop of Permount on slide.

    b. Place coverslip on slide.

1.12 Hematoxylin and Eosin Stain

Reagents

1. Hematoxylin, C.I. 75290
2. Ethyl alcohol
3. Aluminum ammonium sulfate (alum)
4. Mercuric oxide
5. Eosin Y, C.I. No. 45380
6. Potassium dichromate
7. Picric acid (saturated aqueous)
8. Hydrochloric acid
9. Lithium carbonate
10. Xylene
11. Permount

Prepared Reagents

1. Harris' hematoxylin
   a. Prepare Harris' hematoxylin as discussed in Prepared Reagents of Papanicolaou Stain (1.11).
2. Eosin
   a. Place 16 g eosin Y, C.I. No. 45380, in dark glass bottle.
   b. Add 8 g potassium dichromate.
   c. Dissolve eosin and potassium dichromate in 1280 mL distilled water. Warm slightly if required.
   d. Add 160 mL picric acid (saturated aqueous).
   e. Add 160 mL 95% ethyl alcohol.
3. Acid alcohol
   a. Place 650 mL of 70% ethyl alcohol in glass bottle.
   b. Add 1.5 mL hydrochloric acid (concentrated).
4. Lithium carbonate solution
   a. Prepare a saturated solution of lithium carbonate.
   b. Place 1.5 mL of saturated lithium carbonate solution in glass bottle.
   c. Add 650 mL of 70% ethyl alcohol.
5. 95% ethyl alcohol
   a. Prepare 95% solution of ethyl alcohol in distilled water.
6. 80% ethyl alcohol
   a. Prepare 80% solution of ethyl alcohol in distilled water.
7. 70% ethyl alcohol
   a. Prepare 70% solution of ethyl alcohol in distilled water.

Procedure

1. Hydration
   a. 100% ethyl alcohol, 15 dips
   b. 100% ethyl alcohol, 15 dips
   c. 95% ethyl alcohol, 15 dips
   d. 80% ethyl alcohol, 15 dips
   e. 70% ethyl alcohol, 15 dips
   f. Distilled water, 15 dips
2. Chromatin stain
   a. Place in Harris' hematoxylin for 2 minutes.

3. Rinse
   a. Rinse in running tap water until excess stain is removed (approximately 1 minute).
4. Differentiation
   a. Dip 2 times in acid alcohol.
5. Rinse
   a. Rinse in running tap water for 30 seconds.
6. Bluing
   a. Place in lithium carbonate solution for 1 minute.
7. Rinse
   a. Water, 15 dips
   b. 50% ethyl alcohol, 15 dips
8. Counterstain
   a. Place in eosin for 20 seconds.
9. Rinse
   a. Rinse in running tap water until excess stain is removed (approximately 1 minute).
10. Dehydration
    a. 95% ethyl alcohol, 15 dips
    b. 95% ethyl alcohol, 15 dips
    c. 100% ethyl alcohol, 15 dips
    d. 100% ethyl alcohol, 1 minute
11. Clearing
    a. Xylene, 15 dips
    b. Xylene, 15 dips
    c. Xylene, 5–10 minutes
12. Mount
    a. Place 1 drop of Permount on slide.
    b. Place coverslip on slide.

1.13 Test for Fructose (Seliwanoff's)

Reagents

1. Resorcinol
2. Hydrochloric acid

Prepared Reagents

1. Seliwanoff's reagent
   a. Dissolve 50 mg resorcinol in 33 mL concentrated hydrochloric acid.
   b. Dilute to 100 mL with distilled water.

Procedure

1. Place 500 μL (0.5 mL) of semen in test tube.
2. Add 5 mL of Seliwanoff's reagent.
3. Bring to boil.
4. Orange-red color will appear within 1 minute after boiling in presence of fructose. Solution will remain colorless in absence of fructose.

1.14 Test for Fructose (Karvonen and Malm)

Reagents

1. $ZnSO_4 \cdot 7H_2O$
2. NaOH
3. Benzoic acid
4. Indole
5. Fructose
6. Hydrochloric acid

Prepared Reagents

1. 1.8% $ZnSO_4 \cdot 7H_2O$
   a. Prepare 1.8% (w/v) solution of $ZnSO_4 \cdot 7H_2O$ in distilled water.
2. 0.1 M NaOH
   a. Prepare 0.1 M solution of NaOH in distilled water.
3. Indole reagent
   a. Add 200 mg of benzoic acid to 100 mL distilled water.
   b. Dissolve by shaking in 60 °C hot water bath.
   c. Add 25 mg of indole.
   d. Filter and store in refrigerator.
4. Stock fructose standard (2.8 mM)
   a. Dissolve 50.4 mg of fructose in 100 mL distilled water.
   b. Aliquot and store frozen.

5. Working fructose standard
   a. On day of analysis, dilute stock fructose standard to 0.28 mM and to 0.14 mM.

Procedure

1. Add 100 μL (0.1 mL) of semen to 4.9 mL distilled water.
2. Place 1 mL of diluted semen in centrifuge tube.
3. Add 300 μL (0.3 mL) of 1.8% zinc sulfate. Mix.
4. Add 200 μL (0.2 mL) of NaOH. Mix.
5. Incubate at room temperature for 15 minutes.
6. Centrifuge at 2000 g for 20 minutes.
7. Transfer 500 μL (0.5 mL) of supernatant to glass tube with glass stopper.
8. Set up fructose standards in duplicate.
   a. Place 500 μL (0.5 mL) 0.28 mM fructose standard in glass tube with glass stopper.
   b. Place 500 μL (0.5 mL) 0.14 mM fructose standard in glass tube with glass stopper.
9. Place 500 μL (0.5 mL) of distilled water in glass tube with glass stopper to serve as blank.
10. Add 500 μL (0.5 mL) of indole reagent to every tube.
11. Add 5.0 mL of concentrated hydrochloric acid to every tube.
12. Stopper all tubes. Incubate at 50 °C for 20 minutes.
13. Cool in ice water to room temperature.
14. Read color intensity at 470 nm.
15. Calculate fructose concentration (mmol/L)
    a. Fructose mmol/L = $OD_{470 \, nm} \times 75$.
    b. Normal value is 13 μmol or greater.

1.15 Postejaculatory Urine Test

Procedure

1. Immediately after ejaculation, patient should cleanse the penis with water to remove residual semen.
2. Patient should collect urine in clean plastic or glass jar. Care must be taken to include the entire specimen.

3. Transfer the entire urine specimen to centrifuge tubes.

4. Centrifuge urine at 1100 rpm for 10 minutes.

5. Pour off supernatant fluid. Residual fluid adhering to the walls of the centrifuge tubes will provide a small amount of diluent in which to resuspend the sediment.

6. Vortex sediment in all centrifuge tubes.

7. Examine sediment from all tubes using light microscope at 40× magnification.

8. Presence of spermatozoa indicates retrograde ejaculation.

1.16 Bouin's Solution

Reagents

1. Picric acid, saturated aqueous solution (1.2% picric acid in distilled water)

2. Concentrated (36–40%) formalin

3. Glacial acetic acid

Procedure

1. Combine 750.0 mL saturated aqueous solution of picric acid, 250.0 mL concentrated formalin, and 50.0 mL glacial acetic acid. Stir until thoroughly mixed.

2. Store at room temperature.

1.17 Zenker's Solution

Reagents

1. Distilled water

2. $HgCl_2$

3. $K_2Cr_2O_7$

4. Sodium sulfate

Procedure

1. Combine 1000.0 mL distilled water, 50.0 g $HgCl_2$, 250.0 g $K_2Cr_2O_7$, and 10.0 g sodium sulfate. Stir until thoroughly mixed.

2. Store at room temperature.

Bibliography

Adelman MM. Sperm Morphology. Lab Med 1986; 17:32–34.

Amelar RD, Dubin L, Walsh PC. Male infertility. Philadelphia: WB Saunders, 1977:118–132.

Bloom W, Fawcett DW. A textbook of histology. Philadelphia: WB Saunders, 1975:805–857.

Calamera JC, Vilar O. Comparative study of sperm morphology with three different staining procedures. Andrologia 1979;11:255–258.

Coburn M, Wheeler T, Lipschultz LI. Testicular biopsy, its uses and limitations. Urol Clin North Am 1987; 14:551–561.

Cohen J, Edwards R, Fehilly C, et al. In vitro fertilization: a treatment for male infertility. Fertil Steril 1985; 43:422–432.

Dym M. The male reproductive system. In: Weiss L, ed. Histology: Cell and tissue biology. New York: Elsevier Science, 1983:1000–1053.

Eliasson R. Analysis of semen. In: Burger H, deKretser D, eds. The testis. New York: Raven Press, 1981:381–399.

Franklin RR, Dukes CD. Further studies on sperm agglutinating antibodies and unexplained infertility. JAMA 1964; 190:682.

Freund M. Standards for the rating of human sperm morphology. Int J Fertil 1966; 11:97–180.

Hafez ESE. Atlas of human reproduction by scanning electron microscopy. Hingham, Massachusetts: MTP Press, 1982:197–211.

Hafez ESE. Human reproduction conception and contraception. New York: Harper and Row, 1980:91–121.

Hafez ESE. Human semen and fertility regulation in men. St. Louis: CV Mosby, 1976:65–98.

Henry JB. Clinical diagnosis and management by laboratory methods. Philadelphia: WB Saunders, 1979:798.

Jones HW, Jones GS, Hodgen GD, Rosenwaks Z. In vitro fertilization: Norfolk. Baltimore: Williams & Wilkins, 1986:164–167.

Karvonen MJ, Malm M. Colorimetric determination of fructose with indol. Scand J Clin Lab Invest 1955; 7:305–307.

Kibrick S, Belding DL, Merril B. Methods for the detection of antibodies against mammalian spermatozoa. Fertil Steril 1952; 3:430.

Koss LG. Diagnostic cytology and its histopathologic bases. Philadelphia: JB Lippincott, 1979:1211–1230.

Kruger TF, Acosta AA, Simmons KF, et al. New method of evaluating sperm morphology with predictive value for human in vitro fertilization. Urology 1987; 30:248–251.

Lehmann D, Temminck B, DaRunga D, Leibundgut B, Sulmoni A, Muller H. Role of immunologic factors in male infertility. Immunohistochemical and serological evidence. Lab Invest 1987; 57:21–28.

Levin HS. Testicular biopsy in the study of male infertility. Hum Pathol 1979; 10:569–584.

Lynch DM, Leahi BA, Howe SE. A comparison of sperm agglutination and immobilization assays with a quantitative ELISA for anti-sperm antibodies in serum. Fertil Steril 1986; 46:285–292.

Mathur S, Williamson HO, Genco PV, Rust PF, Findenberg HH. Females' isoimmunity to sperm is associated with sperm autoimmunity in their husbands. J Clin Immunol 1985; 5:166–171.

McClure RD. Endocrine investigation and therapy. Urol Clin North Am 1987; 14:480–484.

Mishell Jr DR, Davajan V. Infertility, contraception & reproductive endocrinology. Oradell, NJ: Medical Economics Books, 1986:572–575.

Overstreet JW, Katz DF. Semen Analysis. Urol Clin North Am 1987; 14:446–448.

Pryor JL, Howard SS. Varicocele. Urol Clin North Am 1987; 14:499–511.

Schoysman RJ, Bedford JM. The role of the human epididymis in sperm maturation and sperm storage as reflected in the consequences of epididymovasostomy. Fertil Steril 1986; 46:293–299.

Shulman S. Sperm antigens and autoantibodies: effects on fertility. Am J Reprod Immunol Microbiol 1986; 10:82–89.

Suarez G, Swartz R, Baum N. Male infertility. Postgrad Med 1987; 81:191–198.

Tung K. Immunologic basis of male infertility. Lab Invest 1987; 57:1–4.

Upadhaya M, Hibbard BM, Walker SM. Antisperm antibodies and male infertility. Br J Urol 1984; 56:531–536.

van Lis JMJ, Wagenaar J, Soer JR. Sperm agglutinating activity in the serum of vasectomized men. Andrologia 1974; 6:129.

Wheeler JE, Rudy FR. The testis, paratesticular structures and male external genitalia. In: Silverberg SG, ed. Principles and practice of surgical pathology. Philadelphia: John Wiley and Sons, 1983:1147–1161.

Williams WW. Sterility: the diagnostic survey of the infertile couple. Springfield, Massachusetts: Walter W. Williams. 1964:268–305.

World Health Organization. WHO laboratory manual for the examination of human semen and semen-cervical mucus interaction. NY: Cambridge University Press, 1987:50–51.

Varley H. Practical clinical biochemistry. NY: Interscience Books Inc., 1963:69–70.

Manufacturers

Bristol Laboratories, Evansville, IN 47721.

ELISA kit antisperm antibodies. Universal Diagnostic Systems, Yorktown Heights, New York, 1987.

Penetrak® insert. Serono Diagnostics, Norwell, Massachusetts.

Sigma Chemical Company, PO Box 14508, St. Louis, Missouri 63178.

Spray-Cyte® product instructions. Clay Adams. Becton, Dickenson and Company, Parsippany, New Jersey.

Testsimplets®. Prestained, ready-for-use slides. Boehringer Mannheim GMbH. 6800 Mannheim 31, West Germany.

Index

Numbers in **boldface** refer to pages on which photomicrographs or illustrations appear.

Collection procedures for
spermatozoa, 2, 4–5
coitus to obtain samples
interrupted, 5
uninterrupted, 4, 5
condom used for, 5
masturbation used for, 4
method of collection in container,
4
period of continence in, 2, 4
place used for, 4
Condom, use of, 5
Continence, period of, 2, 4
Cytoplasmic extrusion mass
in midpiece region, 78, **79**
in spermatozoon with absent
acrosome, 48, **49**
in tailpiece, 18, **19**, 22, 48, **49**,
72, **73**

D
Dipsticks containing benzidine
compounds, 6
Dynein arms of spermatozoon
tailpiece, 28, **30**

E
Ejaculate, first fraction of
frequently used for artificial
insemination, 5, 6, 7
prostatic fluid composes, 32
Electrolytes in human seminal
plasma, 33
Electron microscopy of testicular
biopsies, 28–29
ELISA. *See* Enzyme-linked
immunosorbent assay (ELISA)
Endpiece of spermatozoon tailpiece,
14, 16
Enzyme-linked immunosorbent
assay (ELISA)
kit for antisperm antibodies, 114
techniques to detect antibodies to
spermatozoa, 36

Enzymes in human seminal plasma,
34
Eosin-alcohol stain, 102–3
Eosin-nigrosin stain in spermatozoa
viability tests, 40, **41**, 100–101
Eosin Y stain
in hematoxylin and eosin stain,
105–6
in spermatozoa viability tests,
11–12, 40, **41**, 99–100
Epididymal function, 22
Epididymis
anatomy of, 16–17, 29–30
blocked, 30
ducts filled with spermatozoa, 90,
91
Epididymovasostomy, 30
Estrogens, seminiferous tubule
changes resulting from receipt
of, 27
Ethanol abuse as cause of
peritubular fibrosis, 27

F
Fertilization
capacity of semen, factors in, 9
in vitro, 20, 23, 37
Fructose in seminal fluid, 10
test for
Karvonen and Malm, 108–9
Seliwanoff's, 107–8

G
Germ cell. *See* Spermatozoon germ
cell
Germ cell aplasia, 27
Germ cell hypoplasia
(hypospermatogenesis), 27–28
Gonadotropin deficiencies,
postpubertal, 26–27
Guaiac test, 94–95
to determine presence of red
blood cells and/or hemoglobin
in semen specimen, 6

dynein arms, 28, **30**
microtubule doublets, 28, **30**
coiled, 18, **19**, 21–22, 60–63, **61**,
  63, 70–73, **71**, **73**, 80, **81**
curled, 68, **69**, 72, **73**
cytoplasmic extrusion mass, 18,
  19, 22, 48, **49**, 72–75, **73**, **75**,
  78, **79**
endpiece, 14
  flagellar membrane, 16
length, variation in, 18, 21, 68, **69**
  lengthened, 21, 68, **69**
  shortened, 21, 66–69, **67**, **69**
mainpiece (principal piece), 14
  fibrous sheath, 16
  thickness of, 16
midpiece, 14
  abnormality, 18, **19**, 22, 60, **61**,
    74, **75**
  annulus, 16
  kinked, **19**, 22, 60, **61**, 74, **75**,
    78, **79**
  length, 16
  mitochondrial sheath, 16, 22,
    28, **31**
  thickened, 22, 62, **63**, 74, **75**
neckpiece, 14, 16
  cytoplasmic extrusion mass
    accompanies elongated, 22
  lengthened, 18, **19**, 21, 70, **71**,
    80, **81**
  normal, 42, **43**
  thickness of, 14
Sperm count, 7–10, 96–97
  loss of first portion of ejaculate, 4
  multiplied to compensate for
    initial dilution of viscous
    semen, 96
  unilateral obstruction of vas
    deferens, 32
  viscosity of semen and, 7
Sperm density, 7–10, 96–97
Sperm immobilization tests (SIT) to

detect antibodies to
  spermatozoa, 36
Spermine phosphate, 32, 88, **89**
Spermiogenesis, 17, 22
Sperm migration tests, 11, 97–99
Sperm morphology
  analysis of fertilizing capability,
    37
  light microscopy, 18
  principles, 1–37
  procedures, 93–110
  in routine semen analysis, 12
Sperm motility, 97
  in Sertoli cells of seminiferous
    tubules, 16–17, 30
  autoantibodies and isoantibodies
    interfere with, 36
  axoneme responsible for, 28
  coiled tailpiece associated with
    reduced, 22
  determination of, 97
  immotile cilia syndrome results in
    abnormal or absent, 28
  midpiece abnormalities associated
    with reduced, 22
  in routine semen analysis, 10–11
  shortened tailpiece associated with
    reduced, 21
Sperm viability, 11–12
Split-specimen analysis, 4, 5
Spontaneous abortion of in vitro
  pregnancies, 20
Spray-Cyte, 102
Steroid treatment to improve
  fertility in patients with
  antisperm antibodies, 36
Swim-up test of sperm migration, 11
  formula for calculation of, 99
  prepared reagents, 98
  procedure, 97–99
  reagents, 97–98

T
Tailpiece. *See* Spermatozoon
  tailpiece